PSYCHOLOGY PRACTITIONER GUIDEBOOKS

EDITORS
Arnold P. Goldstein, Syracuse University
Leonard Krasner, Stanford University & SUNY at Stony Brook
Sol L. Garfield, Washington University in St. Louis

RATIONAL-EMOTIVE COUPLES THERAPY

Pergamon Titles of Related Interest

Bornstein/Bornstein MARITAL THERAPY:
A Behavioral-Communications Approach

Ellis/McInerney/DiGiuseppe/Yeager RATIONAL-EMOTIVE
THERAPY WITH ALCOHOLICS AND SUBSTANCE ABUSERS

Golden/Dowd/Friedberg HYPNOTHERAPY: A Modern Approach

Meichenbaum STRESS INOCULATION TRAINING

Turner/Beidel TREATING OBSESSIVE-COMPULSIVE DISORDER

Yost/Beutler/Corbishley/Allender GROUP COGNITIVE THERAPY:
A Treatment Method for Depressed Older Adults

Related Journal
(Free sample copies available upon request)

CLINICAL PSYCHOLOGY REVIEW

RATIONAL-EMOTIVE COUPLES THERAPY

ALBERT ELLIS
Institute for Rational-Emotive Therapy

JOYCE L. SICHEL
Private Practice, Dallas

RAYMOND J. YEAGER
Institute for Rational-Emotive Therapy

DOMINIC J. DiMATTIA
University of Bridgeport

RAYMOND DiGIUSEPPE
Institute for Rational-Emotive Therapy

PERGAMON PRESS
New York • Oxford • Beijing • Frankfurt
São Paulo • Sydney • Tokyo • Toronto

Pergamon Press Offices:

U.S.A.   Pergamon Press, Inc., Maxwell House, Fairview Park,
                    Elmsford, New York 10523, U.S.A.

U.K.   Pergamon Press plc, Headington Hill Hall,
                    Oxford OX3 0BW, England

PEOPLE'S REPUBLIC   Pergamon Press, Qianmen Hotel, Beijing,
OF CHINA   People's Republic of China

FEDERAL REPUBLIC   Pergamon Press GmbH, Hammerweg 6,
OF GERMANY   D-6242 Kronberg, Federal Republic of Germany

BRAZIL   Pergamon Editora Ltda, Rua Eça de Queiros, 346,
                    CEP 04011, São Paulo, Brazil

AUSTRALIA   Pergamon Press Australia Pty Ltd., P.O. Box 544,
                    Potts Point, NSW 2011, Australia

JAPAN   Pergamon Press, 8th Floor, Matsuoka Central Building,
                    1-7-1 Nishishinjuku, Shinjuku-ku, Tokyo 160, Japan

CANADA   Pergamon Press Canada Ltd., Suite 271, 253 College Street,
                    Toronto, Ontario M5T 1R5, Canada

Copyright © 1989 Pergamon Press, Inc.

Library of Congress Cataloging in Publication Data

Rational-emotive couples therapy / Albert Ellis . . . [et al.].
    p.   cm. -- (Psychology practitioner guidebooks)
Includes index.
ISBN 0-08-035759-8 -- ISBN 0-08-035758-X (soft)
    1. Marital psychotherapy. 2. Rational-emotive psychotherapy.
3. Cognitive therapy. I. Ellis, Albert. II. Series.
    [DNLM: 1. Marital Therapy--methods. 2. Psychotherapy--
methods. WM 55 R236]
RC488.5.R37   1989   616.89'156--dc19
DNLM/DLC   88-2865
for Library of Congress   CIP

Printed in the United States of America

The paper used in this publication meets the minumum requirements of
American National Standard for Information Sciences -- Permanence of
Paper for Printed Library Materials, ANSI Z39.48-1984

Contents

Chapter 1

RET and Other Theories of Couples Therapy

Cognitive-oriented psychotherapies have achieved great successes in recent years not only in terms of the research and outcome studies which support their effectiveness but also in their increasing public popularity. Their ease in directly treating individual problems makes them more palatable and less threatening than traditional forms of psychotherapy. Also, therapists can often quickly learn to integrate cognitive-behavioral strategies into their armamentarium of therapeutic techniques.

That cognition is a primary factor in human disturbance is not new to the field of psychotherapy. Humans relate and respond to others through the ways they perceive, interpret, and evaluate themselves, their worlds, and their future (Beck, 1976; Ellis, 1957, 1958a, 1960, 1962). Although cognitive therapies more saliently and overtly point this out, most forms of psychotherapy include cognitive features. This chapter illustrates how "competing" schools of psychotherapy try to restructure individual's and couple's belief systems.

A CONJOINT EMPHASIS

When working with couples, therapists are faced with individual disturbances and with the synergistic effect of each individual's problems on the other partner. Therefore, the couple's disturbance is often greater than the mere sum of the disturbances of the individual partners. Rational-emotive couples counseling consequently shares a reciprocal interaction perspective with systems-oriented therapists.

Systems theory holds that individual problems at least partly arise within a family context. Rational-emotive therapy (RET) agrees that your partner's emotions, behaviors, and beliefs serve as activating or influ-

1

encing events for your own problems. Therefore, if you want to minimize your own emotional and behavioral disturbances, you had better change yourself *and* also rearrange your environment *and* the family system in which you live. RET, as Ellis (1985a, 1988a; Ellis & Dryden, 1987) has pointed out, is a form of *double* systems therapy; for it aims to help people change *themselves* within a poor family (or work or social) system, but *also* tries to help them change the *system*.

Let us briefly explain the ABC model of RET. A connotes the Activating Events in people's lives, particularly those (like failure and rejection) that block their goals and desires. C represents their emotional and behavioral difficulties (such as anxiety and self-defeating avoidance). Although people often believe that the Activating Event (A) caused their disturbed Consequences (Cs), Cs are really primarily a function of their Beliefs (B) about the events.

A	Activating Event (e.g., failures, frustrations, rejections).
B	Beliefs about these As.
C	emotional and behavioral Consequences (symptoms or disturbances).

The ABCs of human disturbance are usually expanded as follows:

A	Activating Event (e.g., wife refused to have sex with husband).
rB	rational Belief (e.g., "I wish she wouldn't refuse me. How disappointing. But I can bear her frustrating me and still love her and be happy with her.").
aC	appropriate Consequence (husband feels sad and frustrated but *not* angry or depressed; he keeps trying, subsequently, to have sex with wife).

or

A	Activating Event (e.g., wife refuses to have sex with husband).
iB	irrational Belief (e.g., "She *must* have sex with me when I greatly want it! I *can't stand* her frustrating me! She's a rotten wife and a lousy person!").
iC	inappropriate Consequence (husband feels angry and depressed and refrains from asking for sex for a long period of time).

A couple's disturbed interaction can be structured within the ABC framework when one individual's beliefs, emotions, and behaviors serve as Activating Events for his or her partner, and vice versa. Consider the potential maintenance and circularity of disturbance in the following interaction.

A_1	wife's Activating Events (e.g., husband harshly criticizes her).
iB_1	wife's irrational Beliefs (e.g., "He's being unfair! He *must* not unfairly criticize me like that!").

iC₁   wife's inappropriate emotional and behavioral Consequences (e.g., hurt, anger, withdrawal).

A₂   husband's Activating Events: wife's emotions and behaviors (e.g., wife displays anger and withdrawal).

iB₂   *husband's* irrational Beliefs (e.g., "Too bad I criticized her, but her anger and withdrawal are silly. She *shouldn't* act so childishly!").

iC₂   *husband's* inappropriate emotional and behavioral Consequences (e.g., anger and further criticism of his wife).

A₃   wife's Activating Events (e.g., observation of how angry and increasingly critical her husband is).

iB₃   wife's irrational beliefs (e.g., "My anger at him is only natural and now he unfairly fails to see that and is *more* critical of me than ever. How *horrible* of him to be so doubly unfair!").

iC₃   wife's inappropriate emotional and behavioral Consequences (e.g., increased rage, depression, and withdrawal).

It is important to see this couple's disturbances from an interactional perspective. However, to modify the circularity of their disturbance and the frequent tendency of one of their self-defeating symptoms to encourage the other partner to create irrational Beliefs leading to his or her *own* symptoms, we had better address the Beliefs and the disturbed Consequences of both partners individually *and* collectively. Like Murray Bowen, Nathan Ackerman, and other family therapists, if you want to be an RET couples therapist, you will address individual problems as they arise and maintain the couple's disturbance.

Consider the following example:

A₁   Activating Event: *Husband* is tired after work and expresses disinterest in having sex with his wife.

iB₁   irrational Beliefs: *Wife* expects and *demands* that they have sex more frequently. She *concludes*, "He is either not interested in me or he is having an affair. That is *terrible!*"

iC₁   inappropriate Consequences: *Wife* gets angry and tells her husband that he is "not a man."

A₂   Activating Events: *Husband* observes his *wife's* anger and hears her say he is "not a man."

iB₂   irrational Beliefs: *Husband* demands that his wife be more understanding. "She *must* be nicer! I *can't take* her criticism!"

iC₂   inappropriate Consequences: *Husband* feels angry and hurt and withdraws.

A₃   Activating Events: *Wife* observes her *husband's* anger and withdrawal.

iB₃   irrational Beliefs: *Wife* interprets her *husband's* withdrawal as rejection and believes, "He is unfairly rejecting *me* when *he* is actually at fault! What a worm he is!"

iC₃   inappropriate Consequences: *Wife* gets angry and screams, "You really *are* no good! Sexually and otherwise!"

(and the disturbed interaction spirals downward)

This interaction is clearly both self- and relationship-defeating. The dysfunctional responses (Cs) of one partner serve as Activating Events (As) for the mate. However, these Cs are primarily *caused not by the partner's* behavior but rather by the other's own Beliefs (Bs) about the partner's behavior. If we desire to help change the obnoxious Activating Events (As) for one individual, we had better help the other partner change his or her disturbed Consequences (Cs). And, to arrange this, we would help the first person's partner to change the way he or she *thinks* (B) about his or her original Activating Events (A). Therefore, the RET approach to couples counseling is systems-oriented, like that of the systems therapist. But it also importantly emphasizes specifically understanding and modifying the disturbance-creating Beliefs (Bs) of both individual partners.

As individual disturbances within the couple's system change, more cooperative and more constructive interactions and communications can more readily occur. As stated, the RET couple therapist will examine and show both partners how to change their Belief system (b) in order to make the desired changes in their disturbance. In addition, as will be discussed later in this text, both partners can facilitate cognitive restructuring by acting as a cotherapist for their mates.

Let us now consider various other forms of couples psychotherapy and illustrate how these therapies actually include cognitive themes and how they often use cognitive strategies.

PSYCHODYNAMIC THERAPY

Psychodynamically oriented therapists are often seen as differing radically from rational-emotive therapy and allied cognitive-behavioral therapy (CBT). However, upon close examination, both psychoanalysis and RET see cognition as an important factor in human disturbance.

In reviewing the historical development of RET, we find that Ellis was initially very strongly influenced by such neo-Freudians as Adler and Horney. However, he found that when his psychoanalytic clients significantly improved, they did so largely by making changes in their irrational beliefs. He therefore developed a system of psychotherapy which would more expediently and efficaciously help clients to change their dysfunctional thinking. He also saw that when psychoanalysis works, it indirectly—rather than, as RET does, directly—encourages cognitive change.

Psychoanalysis, for example, often tries to ameliorate the demandingness (in RET terms, the *musts*) of the id and the superego (Ellis, 1962; Wessler & Wessler, 1980). The psychoanalytic view of transference can be seen as cognitive overgeneralization. Thus, a man may demand that *all* women be as nurturing as his mother once was. Or because he thought that his mother was not nurturing *enough*, he may now demand that all people (including his therapist) *should be* more loving. Where, however, the psychoanalyst may help this man *see* his past demands on his mother and on other women, the RET practitioner will help him *rethink* his overgeneralizations and demandingness and *stop* self-defeating transference.

The psychodynamic concept of catharsis can also be translated into cognitive terms. Cognitively oriented therapists hold that catharsis is not beneficial solely because people "get out" or "get in touch with" their feelings. Rather, they hypothesize that, when catharsis works (which it often does not), clients either spontaneously or through direction restructure their self-damning *beliefs* about the material they were previously suppressing. Similarly, holding in one's thoughts and feelings will frequently allow people's irrational beliefs about their past traumas to be maintained.

The RET therapist may encourage couples to reveal their innermost feelings but will also help them understand the Beliefs behind these feelings. Letting couples practice cathartic exercises without showing them how to modify some of their intense disruptive feelings often encourages them to yell and scream at each other without ever learning how to *deal with* these feelings. They often *believe* that violent abreactions are good for them and their relationship. As a result, they are likely to use cathartic expressions *instead of* trying to deal effectively with their interaction problems. Rather than encouraging indiscriminant purging of emotions, the RET therapist helps clients rechannel disruptive emotions and not flood themselves and their partners with them.

SYSTEMS THEORY

Rational-emotive therapy and cognitive-behavior therapy also overlap with several of the family systems therapies (Huber & Baruth, 1989).

Thus, when working with couples, systems therapists find many structural problems. Structural therapists, like Salvatore Minuchin, therefore, seek to reorganize faulty or dysfunctional couples' systems. Although they tend to favor behavioral strategies, cognitive modification is either implied in their strategies or can effectively be utilized along with them.

Couples often present problems when the power hierarchy within the dyad or within the family system is one-sided. One member either assumes too much power or submits too much to the other. These imbalanced roles are typically maintained by one or both partner's *beliefs* that they must be in a superior role or that they are useless and incapable of contributing to the relationship. Similarly, unrealistic *expectations* regarding sex roles may also maintain the misaligned hierarchy. Family-of-origin values and cultural expectations may also predispose a couple to develop and maintain such a disorganized system. The cognitively oriented systems therapist would specifically and directly address these counterproductive Beliefs.

Enmeshment issues are also common in disorganized couples' systems. Partners may be overly involved with their children or with their own parents, thereby violating the "partnership." The Belief that "I must always have the complete love and approval of my parents" or the Belief that "I must always indulge my children" can lead to alienation within the couple's relationship. The RET therapist will work to help both parties challenge and dispute such relationship-defeating notions.

Strategically oriented therapists, such as Jay Haley (1976) and Murray Bowen (1978), can also be viewed within a cognitive framework. Because their focus is typically more on communication as the key to couple disorganization than is the case in the structural therapies, strategic therapists tend to highlight information processing over behavior interactions.

Reframing is perhaps one of the most common therapeutic techniques introduced by strategic therapists. As reframing seeks to restructure a client's dysfunctional perceptions and conceptions, it is clearly cognitive. It typically involves helping clients redefine, relabel (Wells, 1980; Haley, 1976), or recategorize their problems so as to develop a different, more functional perspective. For example, the "bad" fact that a couple comes for treatment may be framed so that they are not hopeless but, rather, that they have the humility and interest to commit to make changes. Setbacks or failures during therapy may also be reframed as learning experiences.

Similarly, the couple's problems can be reframed not as "crazy" or "disturbed" but, rather, as "difficult but understandable." The therapist essentially helps the clients to attach a more productive meaning to their life's activating events. They thereby change the B in the ABC model of RET. Consider the following example of the potentially beneficial effect that reframing procedures may have.

Before reframing:

A   (Activating Event): Couple has a huge fight.
B   (Beliefs): "Our relationship is bad, we obviously do not care at all about each other."

C   (Consequences): Depression, ready to quit on the relationship.

After reframing:

A   Couple has a huge fight.
B   "Our fighting shows that we really do care a great deal about each other. The relationship is so important that we get ourselves 'crazy' about trying to make it perfect. We really do have a lot of love for each other, but just have a bad way of showing it."
C   Motivation to work at making the relationship better.

This example illustrates how a reframing technique modifies the way people can perceive, interpret, and evaluate their relationship problems. They then can take a more relationship-enhancing direction.

BEHAVIOR THERAPY

Behaviorally oriented therapists can benefit by introducing cognitive strategies into their treatment armamentarium so as to facilitate behavior change. Consider the advantages of employing cognitive-restructuring strategies in the following example:

A couple enjoys very little time together, and following a behavior analysis, you (as their therapist) find that they share very few reinforcers. They rarely utilize each other as resources and have become overly independent of each other. What can you do to help this couple?

You can advise these clients to engage in more enjoyable tasks together and go out of their respective ways to bring more "warm fuzzies" (Berne, 1972) into their relationship. You may employ Stuart's (1980) "caring days procedure" to achieve this end.

In cases like this, you may note that this couple may fail to engage in relationship-enhancing procedures because they do not *believe* them to be a viable solution or because they *consider* them to be too difficult. Similarly, this couple may believe that they *should* not have to do reinforcing exercises or that they just *can't*. These and other *beliefs* which prevent couples from taking full advantage of behavior therapy interventions can be modified and restructured in order for effective behavior strategies to be implemented. For techniques such as caring days, graded task assignments, activity scheduling, and contingency contracts to be successful, clients first have to *use* them. Their irrational beliefs and cognitive distortions, however, typically prevent them from fully (or even partly) utilizing them and, therefore, had better be revealed, addressed, and disputed.

Irrationalities may also lead to intense, extreme, and inappropriate emotions which may, in turn, interfere with clients' compliance with behavioral homework assignments. Consider another common example:

> A couple enjoys very little time together, and following a behavior analysis, you, their therapist, find that they actually share very few reinforcers. They rarely utilize each other as resources and have become overly independent of each other. Plus they are very bitter and angry toward each other and frequently fight.

In this example, the couple's difficulties are compounded by extreme emotional reactions (bitterness and anger) which are not only self- and relationship-defeating, but will also likely prevent them from complying with treatment prescriptions. While it is still important to modify their clients' irrational beliefs about the treatment strategies offered, you had better also address the beliefs which cause and maintain their respective bitterness and anger. You will find it next to impossible to get this angry and bitter couple to agree to do "nicey-nicey" with each other when they believe that their partners are no-good blanketty-blanks who deserve to be miserable. Reconstructing the attitudes that go with their anger and bitterness will, therefore, be primary in this couple's treatment.

Obstacles to effective behaviorally oriented treatment are most appropriate grist for the RET mill. Whereas later chapters will more elaborately discuss RET strategies for increasing clients' compliance and cooperation, let us now say that cognitively oriented procedures can be useful, either adjunctively or integrally, for facilitating behaviorally oriented couples therapy.

CLIENT-CENTERED THERAPY

Some couples' counselors prefer to adopt more passive and reflective interventions than are typically used by rational-emotive therapists. However, this need not prevent client-centered counselors from introducing cognitively oriented material into their therapy sessions.

Therapists who prefer to reflect clients' statements and emotions can also reflect their irrational beliefs and cognitive distortions. The RET therapist who chooses to be more passive may reflect to a client: "It sounds to me as if you *need* your husband to be more understanding. Could you tell me more about this *need* for understanding? It sounds as if you are equating *wants* with *necessities*." Socratic dialogue can be used by client-centered and rational-emotive therapists and can be used with a warm, authentic, and reflective style that constitutes a useful therapeutic orientation.

SUMMARY

As can be seen, cognitive strategies already exist with diverse psychotherapeutic schools although they are not made as salient as they are in the more expressly cognitive brands of psychotherapy. Similarly, cognitive elements can be introduced into other forms of counseling to maximize treatment effectiveness. This text will sometimes discuss specific RET and CBT strategies that can be integrated with a therapist's existing noncognitive framework.

Chapter 2
Toward Saner Perspectives on Love and Marital Relationships

> You placed gold on my finger, you brought love like I'd never known. You gave life to our children, and to me a reason to go on. You're my bread when I'm hungry, you're my shelter from troubled winds. You're my anchor in life's ocean, but most of all you're my best friend. When I need hope and inspiration, you're always strong when I'm tired and weak. I could search this whole world over, you'd still be everything that I need.
>
> Popular country-western song recorded by Don Williams (1975, Used by permission of ABC Records, Inc.)

We are a romantic society, for better and worse, and we are American romantics at that—somewhat naive, risk-taking, well-intentioned idealists, who conceive and reach for relationships that will succeed magnificently and fulfill us completely and permanently. We see romantic love as the best reason for marriage and see marriage as the state within which our most significant personal desires will indubitably be satisfied. Despite unignorable evidence to the contrary, we maintain beautifully idealized pictures of wedded bliss. Not for us a mere homestead to provide economic stability, child-rearing, and community participation—not if it's loveless in the romantic sense.

Nor do most of us really want the European's Wednesday night pied-à-terre for sexual and emotional comforts our spouse isn't providing. We are purists—we Americans. It should all be there in the marital package; otherwise we balk. Our consciences prick us to engage in complete honesty. We shudder to think of maintaining convenient, comfortable marriages once "the love is gone." We laugh at our ancestors' arranged marriages, as we try to build "love conquers all" bridges between backgrounds and world views that were never meant to fit together.

We also move away from our parental homes, so that fewer family members will be available to support us. After all, we can take care of each other. We give up same-sex friends for the sake of our mates — truly, shouldn't my spouse also be my closest friend?! And isn't home and marriage a part of religion, too, so that it should take care of our spiritual sides, even as we lessen our involvement with organized religion?!

With these idealistic views, how could our marriages *not* be under strain? To be worth keeping, they are supposed to fill practically all our important desires, apart from work satisfactions. Our spouses had better be exceptionally wise advisors, outstanding emotional supports, and extremely exciting bed partners; have looks that will impress others when we go out together; boost our self-esteem by admiring *us* enormously; instinctively be model parents when that time comes (without, of course, taking any services away from us); age gracefully at the same rate that we do; fully share a satisfying community and social life — and fill any number of additional special "needs" (including neurotic ones) that we may have. Oh, incidentally, our partners had better keep our pulses rushing regularly, too, because romantic love has to last forever; otherwise, whatever else they may provide for us hardly matters.

I (A.E.) described societal fictions about married sex in a book entitled *The American Sexual Tragedy* published back in 1954, especially in a chapter called "The Folklore of Marital Relations." I noted the folly of unrealistic marital expectations:

> It should be obvious to almost any sound-thinking person that while friends, lovers, and business associates are often on their best behavior and consequently will treat one politely and hypocritically, spouses and children are *not* likely to be able to maintain the same kind of urbane pretense for any length of time. . . . Thus, two people who, if they were in the least realistic, would frequently expect the very *worst* kind of behavior from their mates, are quite irrationally asking — nay, demanding — the very best conduct from the other.

I also discussed marital myths in *A Guide to Successful Marriage* (Ellis & Harper, 1961).

A bit later, Lederer and Jackson (1968) pointed out a number of "myths" about marriage that our society held in 1968 and that do not seem to have changed substantially since that time. A. Lazarus (1985) and Beck

(1988) expanded on these marital myths. These are some of the questionable views we tend to hold about marriage:

1. People should marry because they love each other.
2. Nearly all married people continue to be in love with each other.
3. Romantic love is necessary for a satisfactory marriage.
4. There are crucial inherited behavioral and attitudinal differences between males and females.
5. Children automatically improve the potential of a difficult marriage.
6. Loneliness will be cured by marriage.
7. If you ever tell your spouse to go to hell, you have a poor marriage.

Some, but not all, people indoctrinate themselves thoroughly with these myths and hold them devoutly. They take them as gospel — resulting in what RET sees as an *over*valuing of romantic love and an *over*idealization of marriage. These people are the most disturbed when faced with problem-filled reality. They hold highly unrealistic expectations for married life, and often suffer great disillusionment and distress. Norman Epstein (1986, p. 68) presents some unrealistic expectations people commonly hold about relationships: "Disagreement between partners is destructive to the relationship; partners should be able to sense each other's needs and moods as if they could read each other's mind; and partners are not capable of changing."

Perhaps the greatest fiction impeding marital relations is the unrealistic expectation that a really successful marriage just comes naturally — that one doesn't have to try very hard, or make personal sacrifices, or do nice things for our partners beyond the courtship period. No wonder there is so little satisfaction in our marraiges! In this book, we subscribe to the view that people remain in relationships that provide a mutual exchange of satisfactions. In technical terms, this is "social exchange theory," developed by sociologist George Homans (1961) and based on B. F. Skinner's (1953) views of reinforcement.

Viewing relationships as systems of mutual reinforcers may seem less appealing than traditional views of romantic love; however, it is certainly more realistic. It is also much less likely to lead to problems than the fairy-tale expectations about relationships that prevail in our popular culture. Further, social exchange theory is not necessarily the cold-blooded proposition that it may initially seem to be. Enlightened self-interest need not preclude altruistic or loving behaviors. Indeed, RET reflects the principles of ethical humanism, and its notion of "responsible hedonism" suggests that truly rational self-interest incorporates a very real concern for the long-range consequences of one's behavior toward others (Ellis, 1965, 1973a, 1988a; Ellis & Becker, 1982; Walen, DiGuiseppe, & Wessler, 1980).

Historically, marriage was not created primarily to make people happier. It was initially an economic instrument for ensuring the welfare of families, it was a safe and stable environment for raising children, and it was an important unit in church and community participation. It took care of older relatives, and it had continuity, barring deaths, to ensure maximum stability and security in a frequently inhospitable world.

The nuclear family of one set of parents and their children took shape when geographic mobility began to take couples away from their kin and when partners from very different communities could meet and themselves decide to marry without the supports of family and community. As soon as couples were removed from a community context, they looked to each other to make up for whatever was lacking in their lives.

Even in the early 1900s, expectations of marriage were still reasonably low and mainly took the form of avoiding what was quite bad. Common wisdom valued a spouse who was neither alcoholic nor abusive, who brought home a steady paycheck, and who was dependable in times of trouble. These were safety- or security-oriented concerns. Spouses were not required to be sensitive to each other's innermost wishes, to bolster each other's self-esteem, or to be almost continually loving and nicely behaved toward their partner. Lately, couples have added these higher-order expectations to security desires and have come up with a hefty set of societal expectations for marriage, which many people then unfortunately elevate to dogmatic demands because of their disturbed ways of thinking.

So the seeds for marital dysfunction are firmly planted. In a manner similar to bulimics who take society's injunctions to be slim and elevate them into neurotic personal demands, disturbed lovers take societal values about love and marraige overly seriously and elevate them into absolutistic prescriptions. They start with unrealistic expectations and then rigidly demand that their idealistic goals *must* be satisfied.

RET tries to help its clients be saner about romantic love — to be better able to derive love satisfactions but *not* fall victim to love-sickness — a state that Paul Hauck (1977, 1981, 1984) has wisely suggested would be an appropriate psychiatric diagnosis and a state that promotes elaborate courtship rituals to "capture" partners. People who are desperate to fall in love and to have their feelings returned often take sexual attraction for "love" and thereby propel themselves headlong into marriage. "Love" is made into something quite sacred. It is often given *too much* importance and is used as a "good" explanation for some of the most bizarre life choices. Concerns about major discrepancies in background and interests of the partners are frequently ignored—and well-meaning relatives' cautions are seen as unromantic, inappropriately dampening, or even hostile.

Partners think little at the time they marry that their romantic love may eventually fade, yet it most often does, and then they are left to reconcile (if possible) their differing interests, values, and goals to which they were somewhat blind earlier. In the disillusionment of finally seeing one's partner realistically, people again often follow "love's dictates" and reject this person completely. If he or she is not one's *true* love, you can legitimately find him or her *worthless* (Ellis, 1977a; Ellis & Harper, 1961).

Since there are so many things a modern marriage partner can provide, and the culture encourages us to aim high, each of us at any given time will have a laundry list of desires—at least partly societally determined. We may think of accepting less as "settling," in the worst sense of the word, if (for example) we select someone who is not both a *Playboy* bunny and a Rhodes' scholar. We may think of our marriage as "lousy" if it lacks any of the assets near the top of our laundry list. And we may rather quickly dispose of an imperfect marriage and try again for "the real thing" a second or third time around.

Frequently there are developmental stresses in the life of a union—from adjusting to the realities of living with another person, to adjusting to babies, children, and adolescents, to launching the children and living with each other again, to accepting the changes of aging. We expect the same union to survive resiliently through all these changes—and preferably without professional help. It is more realistic to expect a marriage to work well for a limited peroid of time. To expect otherwise is to assume static individuals who experience little growth as adults, or to predict that two distinct individuals will somehow grow in complementary ways.

Other strong evidence for our society's extreme romanticism is the frequency with which people get addicted to love. Either we are hooked on loving a single individual who we are "sure" will give us our heart's greatest desires, or we get hooked on the highs of being in love—regardless of the object. Dorothy Tennov (1979) has written about "limerence," an extreme obsessive-compulsive type of love to which certain people are highly susceptible. We don't tend to see it as the sickness it really is, since it is so much a part of our literature and theater. But this form of love produces psychological cravings and withdrawal symptoms much like other addictions. Social psychologist Stanton Peele (1976) was probably the first to really call it an addiction and to believe that it is a response to fear: "disbelieving his own adequacy . . . the addict welcomes control from outside himself as the ideal state of affairs" (p. 55).

Wanderer & Cabot (1978) have also written about love addictions which they conceptualize as reflections of "attachment hunger"—left over from being poorly loved in childhood. Sometimes people who are intensely involved with each other are really engaged in neurotic folie à deux. Although usually *not* rooted in childhood deprivation, but in the irrational belief that one absolutely *must* be adored by parents, siblings, and practically everyone else, obsessive-compulsive love can involve getting the better of a partner, wringing "love" out of a stingy mate, or any number of other loveless, desperately played games where the stakes are seen as crucial—self-esteem, happiness, and perhaps even survival. "I love him but I can't stand him" is often a clue to this unhealthy kind of "love" that is really much more like an addiction.

Disturbed thinking is often even more evident in regard to *loss* of love. All kinds of human cruelty and insane acts have been committed in the name of jealousy and despair about lost love. In our culture, it is considered appropriate to be quite possessive of a mate. Jealousy (if not taken to unusual extremes) is seen as flattering and desirable. The loss of a love is considered a good reason for deep and protracted depression, since it is so often accompanied by lowered self-esteem. And because often the love partnership is the primary (even only) source of hope for life satisfaction, suicides and homicides in the wake of lost love often seem understandable although tragic (Ellis, 1984a; Tennov, 1979).

In the interests of bringing greater sanity to the experiences of love and marriage, we invite readers (and therapists!) to entertain seriously a relatively hard-nosed approach to this tender area. We believe that it is humanistic to strengthen people's reason so that it balances or minimizes their disturbed emotions. Hence, the term "rational-emotive" theory and therapy.

RET teaches that the most disturbed individuals—those who are often seen in marital therapy—elevate marital preferences to needs and demands, vastly exaggerate the disadvantages they have in their marriages, convince themselves that they cannot stand their less than perfect situations, and make themselves furious at those who imperfectly provide for their "needs" (Ellis, 1954, 1973a, 1977a, 1988a; Ellis & Harper, 1961, 1975).

Cognitions—in the form of values, expectations, and preferences—are socially encouraged and produce many people's marital goals. But social standards also encourage much interpersonal misunderstanding and conflict between marital partners. In addition, they frequently encourage one spouse to blame his or her feelings and behavior on the other. Thus, many people enter marital therapy accusing their *partner* of causing their own disturbances. If you want to practice as an RET marital therapist, you will want to know not only what each partner is supposedly *doing* to "upset" the other, but also what each has been *thinking* about the other. Remember that RET hypothesizes that crooked thinking contributes enormously to marital disturbance.

Do modern Americans' thoughts about love, marriage, and their mates amount to pure nonsense? No, but they include much nonsense that you can help correct through a rational-emotive approach. We would certainly support those who wish to get many of their desires satisfied in a close, loving relationship. It is wonderful to have someone we deeply care for also care for us and look out for our interests. It is often worth working hard to develop this kind of intimate relationship.

However, to insist that one close relationship be the perfect union — to demand that all our desires be met through it — is almost going to guarantee marital turmoil, just as insisting that we cannot be happy at all without love will practically ensure personal disturbance. The rational-emotive (R-E) approach encourages *desiring* without *demanding* that a primary relationship give us what we want, building up our tolerance for inevitable mating frustrations and avoiding blowing things out of proportion when they do not go well. RET encourages nondemanding and unangry ways of responding to our partners, though it often favors firmness.

In the practice of RET, you also encourage clients to be more realistic and less gullible in subscribing to societal myths. You help them examine their previously unexamined values and assumptions — some derived from subcultures and some from idiosyncratic family systems (especially from highly disturbed families) — to see if they actually make sense and lead to satisfying living.

RET also supports those who are not highly interested in love relationships, or who choose an atypical life-style, such as devotion to work or to a cause. It helps clients resist some social pressures. It also helps people avoid undue sentimentalizing, to stop sacredizing their emotions, and not to take themselves and their marital lives overly seriously.

While Americans have often too hastily resorted to divorce, they have at other times foolishly clung to highly unsatisfying matings out of a belief that marriage is holy and has to be preserved at almost all costs. This was truer early in our century, but is even true today among some groups. Marital counselors may even abet this philosophy by adopting a mission of "saving marriages" rather than maximizing the happiness of the couples involved.

The next chapter will expand this theme.

Chapter 3
Rational-Emotive Theory of Relationship Disturbance

Disturbed feelings and behaviors in relationships are not merely caused by one's mate's wrongdoing or from other adverse events. The partners themselves largely *create* or *construct* their disturbance in the wake of these provocations. The rational-emotive theory (RET) states that mates are directly disturbed not by each other's actions, or by life's rough breaks, but rather by the views they take of these actions and breaks. Thus, RET focuses on the *individuals* in the relationship—they are considered to be the main focus of disturbance rather than *only* their interactions or *only* the system in which they exist. RET is always concerned with couples' feelings and actions, but especially with the *thinking* in which each partner engages. It is this thinking that largely leads to anger and the other disturbed emotions and interactions between marital partners.

The relationship between thought and emotion and behavior is strong and dependable, but some psychologists still argue about whether thinking is a *necessary* prerequisite to emotional experience (R. Lazarus, 1982, 1984; Zajonc, 1980, 1984). RET theory holds that thinking, feeling, and acting are quite interactional and that each of these processes continually influences and affects the other two (Ellis, 1958a, 1962, 1987d, 1988a; Ellis & Dryden, 1987). Most psychologists now agree that thinking importantly interacts with emotional states and greatly intensifies feelings.

"Irrational" thinking, we believe, frequently produces both personal neurosis *and* relationship disturbance. By "irrational" we mean thinking that is highly exaggerated, inappropriately rigid, illogical, and, especially, absolutist. People can usually perceive, interpret, and evaluate the events in their relationships more or less rationally. When they think *ir*rationally, they tend to lose their perspective and to command, like

17

grandiose children, that things *must* be different from what they are. Since they have such limited control over their spouses and the events of their lives, they quickly create their own misery in the face of less than perfect reality (Ellis, 1957, 1958b, 1962, 1973a, 1988a; Ellis & Dryden, 1987; Ellis & Harper, 1961, 1975).

One of us (A.E.) developed the RET ABC theory of human disturbance, which, as noted earlier, helps therapists and their clients understand how events play only a limited role in human disturbances. Let us suppose that a man's wife nags him considerably. We can call her nagging an Activating Event (A) for this man and agree it is hardly pleasant to live with. Because it blocks his goals (e.g., peace and comfort), and he *prefers* her nagging to stop, his preference produces an appropriate feeling or Consequence (C) of displeasure or disappointment.

However, let us suppose that the man is much more than displeased with his wife's nagging. He views it as the worst behavior that anyone could suffer and devoutly believes that she *must* not, under *any* condition, keep nagging him. This is his absolutist evaluation or irrational Belief (iB) about the event. Holding this commanding irrational Belief, he will almost inevitably experience highly inappropriate and disturbed Consequences. He will probably be furious at her and disposed to express his rage in some violent manner. Perhaps he will yell or act sarcastically (behavioral Consequence). People in relationships are sometimes ready to kill each other. Their hostile thoughts and feelings impel hurtful actions unless checked by counterbalancing, mature, self-helping thoughts (Ellis, 1977a).

What are the major kinds of irrational thinking that lead to extreme states of distress? They can be grouped in terms of "demandingness," "neediness," "intolerance," "awfulizing," and "damning" kinds of beliefs. Let us try to capture the flavor of each.

DEMANDINGNESS

The most fundamental irrationalities about relationships derive from a philosophy of *requiring* as opposed to *desiring*. People naturally and easily slip into requiring things of themselves, others, and the environment, rather than preferring (however strongly) that certain things be present in their relationships. When you dogmatically require certain features or behaviors from a partner, you almost inevitably will feel angry, cheated, or self-pitying when your requirements fail to be fulfilled. If, for example, you demand that your mate be unfailingly supportive (despite your own inevitable imperfection), you are likely to be frequently outraged by less than complete support. Your irrational Beliefs are most revealingly shown by *should* or *must* statements you carry in your head about relationships in general and your own in particular: "Partners *should* be completely supportive!" "Spouses *must* always put each other first!" "My mate *should* be completely sensitive to what I want!" Et cetera. Examining these implicit requirements usually shows that you believe them rigidly — even though you also have more rational beliefs which reflect your understanding that human partners cannot be expected to unfailingly support each other (Ellis, 1962, 1971, 1973a, 1988a).

Dogmatic *shoulds* about your partner's actions and feelings are prime targets for change in marital therapy. Your rigid requirements are likely to produce *in*appropriate, disturbed feelings, while your strong preferences or values, when you do not add musts and commands, tend to produce appropriate feelings of frustration, disappointment, and regret.

Your expectancies about relationships may be held demandingly or preferentially, and both demands and preferences may be weak or strong. Even a realistic preference or probabilistic expectation (e.g., for moderately frequent sexual relations in marriage) may be held highly demandingly. Thus, you may tell yourself, "I *must* always have at least a moderate amount of sex in my marriage, and if my mate doesn't give it to me, he or she is no damned good!" Your "moderate" demand, then is *still* likely to produce personal and relationship disturbance. And, conversely, an unrealistic desire (e.g., for a wife to iron a husband's underwear like his mother did) may be held *non* demandingly and cause few problems (Ellis, 1985a, 1985b, 1987a, 1987b).

In dysfunctional marriages, partners may demandingly hold more than the usual number of desires about a spouse's behavior and the nature of the marriage. Disturbed spouses' desires may be highly unrealistic because they have not been modfied in the light of early marital experience. Demandingness has been retained even in the face of starkly contradictory reality (undemandingly held unrealistic desires are far more likely to be modified by disconfirming evidence), for demanding beliefs and attitudes color people's perception of reality and the inferences that are made about it. In terms of the RET model, Activating Events are filtered through a sieve of Beliefs. They are created by people as well as existing in their environment.

While idealistic thinkers may warm themselves by beautiful pictures they cherish in their hearts, they are also likely to hold in their heads the most irrational beliefs about how relatinships *must* be. Real relationships, no matter how good, rarely correspond to such idealized views.

You also frequently hold rigid requirements about yourself in a relationship — "I *must* succeed (especially if I failed before)!" "I *must* win total and constant love!" "*I must* easily handle my partner's difficult behavior!" "*I must* be able to make this relationship work!" When your commands apply mainly to your self, you are usually less angry at others but more likely to be anxious and depressed. In your relationships, you tend to see yourself falling short of your goals of perfect success or control of others, and your confidence and security are thus threatened (Ellis, 1962, 1977a, 1988a).

NEEDINESS

People often convince themselves that they absolutely require certain things — for any happiness in life and for feeling good about themselves. By creating a dire need for love (either from some special person or from many others), many otherwise functional people make themselves crazy. They become highly anxious about getting their love supplied (much as an addict would) and become quite withdrawn and depressed when the love they believe they absolutely require is not completely forthcoming (Ellis, 1976a, 1979a).

In relationships, irrational neediness tends to lead to extreme jealousy and possessiveness. The value that society gives to love is personally elevated to an importance almost equal to that of air and water (Ellis, 1954, 1972a, 1984a).

Sometimes irrational Beliefs reflect requirements seen as essential for future happiness: "My happiness depends solely on keeping my partner's love!" "I must make this relationship work because it's my last chance!" "I'll never find another person this wonderful!" "I should be able to guarantee that this relationship will last forever!"

Requirements, often pernicious for mental health, are tied to the relevance of a relationship to self-worth. People believe they *need* to be lovingly mated because otherwise they are worthless. What they fail to realize is that they would be *making themselves* "worthless" if they lost their relationship. It is only *they* who invent the equation between being loved and being worthy (Ellis, 1972b, 1977c, 1979a).

LOW FRUSTRATION
TOLERANCE

People also irrationally convince themselves that they *can't stand* the problems they experience or anticipate in their relationships. Fear of being "hurt,"' so common in relationships, often stems from the belief that really bad feelings are intolerable — that one *shouldn't* have to suffer such feelings. Couples childishly insist that they not have to risk frustration when trying for a satisfying relationship. Once people have a history of being "hurt," they focus on a possible repetition, convince themselves they couldn't stand it, and come to dread the possibility. They thereby make themselves overly anxious and hypervigilant.

"Discomfort anxiety," as RET calls it, surfaces strongly when mates have friction and insist that they *should* have fewer hassles or that their partner *must* be less of a pain in the ass. "This is so bad, I simply *can't stand* it! It's more than a nice person like me *should* have to bear!"

People with low frustration tolerance (LFT) often think like perpetual victims: "My partner makes my life too hard for me! Life should give me a better shake since I try so hard (or give the most)!" Couples create trouble by demanding a relationship with only gentle treatment and no major problems. But those who react nonassertively to problems will tend to feel self-pity, depression, and "confirmed" victimization. They may additionally feel intolerance for life's inherent unfairness. "Victims" may take the societal myths about perfect love and riding off into a sunset (without working on one's relationship) overseriously. They dwell mentally in fairy tales and often need help to tolerate imperfect human realities and the normal unfairness of life (Ellis, 1972c, 1978, 1979b, 1980a).

AWFULIZING

Requiring certain things in a relationship and being intolerant of variations often results in *awfulizing* and *catastrophizing* when things are not all they are *supposed* to be. Awfulizers believe that it is not merely very bad but *more than* bad — *awful!* — when their partner is not giving ideally. Or they feel that it is *terrible* (badder than it *should* be) that they have not won perfect love or succeeded in some total and guaranteed way. Or *horrible* (full of *horror*) that the relationship has problems. This kind of thinking exaggerates the badness of an unfortunate situation — ironically adding to the person's distress (Ellis, 1973a, 1988a; Ellis & Becker, 1982; Ellis & Dryden, 1987; Ellis & Harper, 1975).

DAMNING OF ONESELF OR OTHERS

Destructive ways of thinking that are likely to lead to chronic distress in a relationship, to undermining of confidence, and sometimes to desperation (and even suicide or homicide) occur when people's personal value is tied to how their relationship is going. Commonly, they define themselves as worthless if their partner does not appear to value them enormously (and to prove it constantly). The partner's feelings are taken as a mirror of one's lovability and human value—with little realization that the two do not have to be equated. This kind of conditional thinking about self-worth is especially prevalent among jealous partners—who seem to be seeking to validate their personal worth by trying to assure that their mate is faithful. They make their stake in relationship success overwhelming, because they insist that the survival of their personal integrity depends on it. Clients will literally tell their therapist that they are less than whole people without their partner's complete attention. They also often feel enraged and vindictive when their partners "sabotage" their self-esteem by being less loving than they *should* be (Ellis, 1972a; 1984a).

Also crippling is the perfectionistic demand to succeed at an important relationship. People irrationally believe that they can be worthy only if they win their would would-be partners. Especially when they have a history of failures at relationships, they may strongly put themselves down if they have another failure. They may anxiously try to gain insurance against failure—putting much pressure on themselves and their partners—and may easily become depressed by their futile need for certainty. These kinds of conditional self-ratings (instead of unconditional self-acceptance) produce much anxiety in relationships. Self-rating also leads to defensive maneuvers to protect one's self-image that is seen to be so easily in danger (Ellis, 1972b, 1973a, 1979a).

Labeling one's partner as "a rotten person" is another result of damning thinking. This, again, is foolish overgeneralization—an illegitimate leap from specific dissatisfactions to condemning the partner as a whole. It is like the "splitting" phenomenon noted in "borderline" personalities. These individuals rate others as either all good or all bad. Much cruelty in intimate human relations is, of course, inspired by "all-bad" labeling.

If relationships are troubled because couples disturb themselves with irrational ideas, the RET therapist's task is to expose and help them change their major irrationalities. Demandingness is thereby eased into desiring, neediness is abated, higher frustration tolerance is built, awfulizing is deawfulized, and damning of self and others is halted (Ellis, 1962, 1971, 1973a, 1988a; Ellis & Harper, 1961, 1975).

Because RET favors a social exchange approach to marriage, we are also concerned with the level of *satisfaction* as well as the level of *disturbance* in a relationship. If marital satisfaction mainly derives from the trade in rewarding behaviors, partners may be merely dissatisfied with what they are getting and also may be disturbed *about* their lack of satisfaction. The RET approach to marital dysfunction often focuses on marital *disturbance*, but also strongly attempts to achieve couple *satisfaction*. Using RET, you discover how clients' irrational Beliefs bring about their individual disturbances and also create needless partnership dissatisfactions.

Relationship dissatisfaction, however, may stem from rational preferences rather than from irrational demands. People *sensibly* may ask that a relationship be more rewarding than it is. Dissatisfactions may occur for any number of reasons, some of which have little to do with psychopathology, deep-seated conflicts, or irrational demands by either partner.

As we pointed out earlier, people's notions about what is or is not satisfying may change over time, simply in the course of normal human development. A relationship that was considered very satisfying when a couple were in their twenties may seem less so once the partners, who have developed new interests and pursuits over the years, move into their forties. Also, a mate who was considered the best choice at one time may come to seem less satisfying if the partner's alternatives widen to include more desirable potential mates. A person's choice of mate may also have been less than satisfactory to begin with and become worse through the years.

Whatever the cause of relationship dissatisfaction, it may involve negative feelings that, though they be quite intense, are nonetheless appropriate. People who are rationally dissatisfied because their partner does not provide what they want in a relationship will experience such emotions as sadness, disappointment, annoyance, regret, or concern rather than necessarily feeling inappropriately and dysfunctionally depressed, angry, guilty, or panicked (Ellis, 1977a, 1977b, 1977c, 1979a; Ellis & Harper, 1975). Their behavior, too, may be quite adaptive. They may try to improve the relationship by various means, or if improvement is not feasible, they may attempt to make the best of an apparently bad bargain or decide to leave the marriage.

Problems that involve *relationship disturbance*, on the other hand, usually stem from irrational *needs* or *demands* (on the part of one or both partners) that a relationship be other than it manifestly is. The couple will tend to have intense, inappropriate feelings like severe anxiety, rage, guilt, and depression, and will promulgate maladaptive actions that will tend to escalate their difficulties. Disturbance thus "turns up the volume" on whatever troubles the couple experience and often becomes an additional source of dissatisfaction with the relationship.

As the foregoing paragraphs suggest, relationship dissatisfaction need not lead to relationship disturbance. Partners may be quite dissatisfied with a relationship and still not become disturbed or neurotic about the situation unless they create and maintain irrational Beliefs about it. On the other hand, we hypothesize that relationships disturbances will almost always demote marital satisfaction.

RET goes beyond behavioral approaches that mainly provide understanding of marital satisfiers and dissatisfiers. It distinguishes between rational wants (e.g., not based on dire needs for love and attention) and irrational demands (e.g., based on dire needs for success and comfort). It also discovers whether there is a reasonably rational (tolerant and nondamning) response to the wants or demands of one's partner.

Equity in what one is giving and getting in relationships is largely a matter of subjective judgment. What seems fair to one person may seem manifestly unfair to another, and individuals may hold widely different views as to how much or what kind of reinforcement it is fair to expect in a relationship. People's definitions of equity, and their consequent tendency to perceive given situations as just or unjust, often follow from their general belief system. For example, people with a dire need for love may consider it grossly unfair when their partners fail to provide continuous affection, where those with a desire but no demand for love may perceive minimal affection as merely unfortunate or unpleasant. Similarly, individuals with low frustration tolerance may complain that their partner is unfair whenever they do not get what they want, and especially when they do not get it immediately.

LFT, or discomfort anxiety, is a major source of perceived inequity in relationships. Most relationships are best (that is to say, rationally) evaluated as equitable or inequitable over the long haul rather than in the short run. Temporarily "inequitable" situations may be willingly tolerated by partners who view them as compromises that will enable the couple eventually to achieve certain long-term goals. One partner, for example, may be willing to tolerate putting off his or her individual plans for starting a career or a family, to put the other through school, or a partner who is temporarily unable to give a great deal of attention to the relationship while completing an important work project may give up certain pleasures in order to help the other mate in some way. In relationships like this, there is a long-term "accounting system" for balancing the couple's resources, and the partners generally trust each other eventually to reimburse temporary frustrations rather than (so to speak) abscond with the funds. Such arrangements reflect a high degree of frustration tolerance and a rational philosophy of long-range hedonism.

People with LFT, on the other hand, characteristically maintain an irrational philosophy of short-range hedonism and tend to operate on a quid pro quo basis in their relationships. They typically demand that the equity of the relationship be evaluated immediately after every transaction and insist that the books balance perfectly (or in their favor) every time. If at any given instant this is not the case, they frequently scream for an audit and start hurling accusations of foul play, which they often follow up with an attempt to coerce their partner into immediately repaying whatever debt they irrationally believe is "owed." Their coercive behaviors may well result in diminished satisfaction for their mate and may bring about reprisals which clients with LFT will define as even more unfair and intolerable than actually is true (Ellis, 1976b, 1977a, 1979b, 1980a).

In maintaining that marital disturbance stems primarily from both partners' disturbances rather than from the "system" the partners share, RET differs markedly from many theories of family therapy. However, it recognizes the interactive nature of family members' irrational thinking and behaving, and it theorizes that individual disturbance is most likely to lead to marital disturbance when a partner provides those activating events that will easily trigger the other's irrational thinking and behaving. One partner's belief system can actually be quite irrational, but cause minimal relationship problems if the person has chosen a mate with similar or complimentary irrationalities ("the rocks in his head fit the holes in hers").

Thus, a spouse's judgmental attitude, even involving several demands about how the partner "must" be, may not upset a mate who is self-confident and assertive. However, the same critical demands may lead to emotional havoc when the mate is highly sensitive to criticism and irrationally believes that he or she must be perfect and always win approval. In this case, the demander's criticism will encourage the vulnerable partner to become defensive and perhaps completely withdraw.

David Burns (1984) has been factor analyzing numerous attitudes that he believes cause distress when they interact with another partner's beliefs. Some kinds of irrational thinking patterns, like a highly blaming attitude, he finds, almost always create relationship disturbance. In such cases we are dealing with demandingness that RET also sees as sources of marital problems. RET particularly deals with demandingness, and the anger to which it leads, in marriage problems, as illustrated in the verbatim excerpts from a rational-emotive therapy session, as shown in Chapter 11 of *A Guide to Personal Happiness* (Ellis & Becker, 1982).

Chapter 4
General Clinical Issues

Unlike many approaches to marital therapy, the rational-emotive approach views the individual partners as the clients—the relationship is important but secondary to their happiness as people. What is good for one or both of the individuals may not be good for their relationship, and vice versa. Robert Harper (1981, p. 5) has sounded this RET keynote: "I see my role as one of helping each individual in these relationships to function less self-defeatingly, more creatively, and more happily." The RET therapist's main agenda, then, is to save people first—and also, perhaps, to save their marriages. Nor are RET therapists obsessed with changing a couple's "system," although they are very interested in how spouses specifically iteract and how they can better interrelate.

In subscribing (though not dogmatically) to the social exchange theory of marriage, RETers are interested, especially for assessment purposes, in the kinds of exchanges in which a particular marital couple is involved. Using RET, you will probably want to see the individuals conjointly some of the time, but you need not have any overriding commitment to conjoint sessions.

In assessing *dissatisfaction* problems, you may often spend some time with each partner separately. While this practice is often discouraged in couples therapy, because it may arouse fears about what is going on in each partner's individual session, the risks of *not* having any separate sessions may be substantial. Often, information that clients *don't* disclose in a conjoint session is more important for a valid assessment of the problem (and, in turn, effective treatment of the problem) than what they *do* reveal. By seeing the couple only in conjoint sessions, you risk remaining ignorant of infidelities, lies, complaints, and individual agendas that the spouses may be unwilling to disclose in the presence of their partners.

Differences in the degree of irrationality and emotional upsetness may also encourage you to see the mates separately, and sometimes to recommend more intensive individual work for one of the partners. Conjoint sessions tend to be most helpful when you can spend approximately equal amounts of time working with the disturbance of each client. This is important in ensuring that you are not perceived as singling out one partner as more disturbed, and as thereby somehow taking sides.

When one partner clearly does seem to be more disturbed than the other, unbalanced conjoint sessions may encourage more resistance and defensiveness than they do positive change. In such cases, it may thus be preferable to see the clients separately, at least for a brief period, to allow you to give more time and attention to disputing the more disturbed person's irrational Beliefs (iBs).

Given that a successful marriage relationship is a challenge even for healthy individuals, if one partner is distinctly disturbed, there is likely to be marital dysfunction. He or she will tend to respond anxiously or angrily even to relatively normal frustrations and to the partner's sensible requests. When the marital life situation includes extreme problems, the disturbed individual will usually overreact more severely. And if *both* marital partners are disturbed, the interaction between them easily leads to mutual temper tantrums.

Separate individual sessions may also be preferable when both partners are so angry that their conjoint sessions serve as an opportunity to exchange verbal vitriol. So by all means be flexible! Although you may generally prefer seeing both partners together, you can feel free to see them separately when a specific case seems to call for it.

When disturbance arises intrapersonally and/or interpersonally, rational-emotive theory holds that it can be traced back to the interaction of people's irrational cognitions with their sensory, emotional, and behavioral processes (Ellis, 1962, 1973a, 1981, 1982; Ellis & Dryden, 1987; Ellis & Grieger, 1977, 1986; Ellis & Harper, 1975; Ellis & Whiteley, 1979).

Consequently, the meat and potatoes of the rational-emotive therapist's work are the thinking patterns of the clients, and the focus for treating marital disturbance is heavily cognitive, as well as emotive and behavioral. You may spend a substantial amount of time assessing the clients' styles of irrational thinking (e.g., demandingness, awfulizing, overgeneralizing, and damning). You teach them how they themselves (and not their mates) largely cause their own disturbance. You help them take the main responsibility for overcoming their self-destructive, marriage-damaging ideas. You teach them how to question and challenge unrealistic, illogical, and self-defeating attitudes. We call this process *Disputation* or *Disputing*. It represents the "D" stage in the ABC model. A more rational *Effective New Philosophy* ("E") is aimed for, to help clients deal with troublesome issues more logically and less extremely. You also spend time on the content of thinking as well as its style. The nature of the partners' expectancies and their attributions about each other's behavior are targeted for scientific inquiry and challenging.

Using behavioral methods, which the RET therapist combines extensively with cognitive methods, you may ask couples to role play, to take deliberate risks, and to do what is awkward and difficult (e.g., keep their mouths shut when tempted to criticize their partners). Rational-emotive couples therapy stresses activity homework assignments and favors their being done in vivo rather than only in the couples' imagination. It encourages couples, in many instances, to remain together even though they may currently find it unpleasant, until they have worked on their destructive thoughts and feelings and learned not to unduly upset themselves (Ellis, 1957, 1975a, 1975b, 1987c, 1988b; Ellis & Becker, 1982; Ellis & Harper, 1961, 1975).

Using RET, you often employ reinforcement methods that include having partners contract with each other, so that one agrees to help the other in some way (e.g., by communicating better) while the other agrees to do something the first one wants (e.g., keeping expenses under better control). You may also offer considerable skill training, such as teaching couples how to be more assertive or to have better sex relations. You often help them do practical problem solving and to look objectively at relationship's costs and balances. Humor is often employed to help the partners gain perspective on their problems. Your language may, but need not necessarily, be dramatic or even shocking to stir clients' emotional responses and help shake them out of habitual patterns (Dryden, 1984; Ellis, 1977d, 1977e, 1987d; Ellis & Dryden, 1987).

You will often show clients how to practice behavioral management of couples' in-session problems, especially in conjoint sessions. Clients are discouraged from spending much time arguing with each other. Ground rules are sometimes set that call for terminating sessions when this behavior continues. The partners may be seen separately for a while until their anger has been worked on and reduced.

Ethically, we realize that we can significantly influence people's lives. So try to be sure that all decisions are made by the clients and truly owned by them. Attempt to unblock all routes that couples close by their irrational thinking. Do not knowingly open one pathway but leave another important alternative closed. For example, not only try to help people overcome intense guilt that prevents them from leaving their marriage, but also work on their low frustration tolerance that exacerbates their marital dissatisfaction.

Once major blocks are removed, let your clients' preferences and values override your own. What is satisfying or pleasurable is a highly individual matter, and one that is subject to change over time. Rational-emotive therapy sees a good relationship as one that provides a great deal of flexibility. It posits no absolute standards for what people should or should not do individually and as couples. Indeed, the main thrust of RET is to try to reduce the emotional and behavioral dysfunctions stemming from absolutistic thinking, particularly from unconditional *shoulds, oughts, musts,* and other forms of dogmas (Ellis, 1957, 1962, 1971, 1985a, 1985b, 1987a, 1988a; Ellis & Becker, 1982; Ellis & Dryden, 1987; Ellis & Grieger, 1977, 1986). However, RET respects clients' *preferences* —even if their preferences are unpopular with their family or friends (or therapist!).

Whether people choose conventional or less conventional styles of relating, try to free them to make choices that are not based on gullibility about marital myths, on rigidly held life philosophies, or on panic-induced avoidance.

The basic idea that there are no absolute or uniform prescriptions for good relationships is easier to acknowledge than to accept and carry into practice, and we often find in supervising rational-emotive couples therapy that we have to work with therapist's beliefs. Therapists, like other humans, have their own personal preferences and values and may also have developed specific ideas as to what constitutes psychologically healthy relationships. If, like other fallible humans, they transmute their rational beliefs into irrational ones about mating, a variety of problems can (and often do) arise (Ellis, 1985a).

When therapists maintain irrational Beliefs about relationships that coincide with those of one or both clients, therapeutic effectiveness can be seriously impaired. Suppose, for example, a therapist shares a client's irrational Belief that it *would* indeed be awful if Mrs. X. engaged in extramarital affairs or if Mr. Y. attempted to thwart his wife's desires to develop her career interests. Such therapists had better recognize and vigorously dispute their own irrational Beliefs as a first step toward helping clients do the same.

Another kind of problem can arise when therapists escalate their own preferences, values, and pet psychological theories about good relationships into absolutistic prescriptions for client behaviors. The therapist who irrationally demands, for example, that "Mr. and Mrs. Z. learn to communicate openly and honestly" will probably feel inappropriate and untherapeutic anger when the couple persists in communicating "badly."

Further, demands that clients adopt the therapist's views can lead to unethical counseling. RET practitioners, therefore, work hard at accepting *clients* but not their *irrationalities* and at accepting clients' rights to maintain their own relationship values, however different these may be from those of the therapist.

Using RET with couples, you try to assist the partners — via cognitive, emotive, and/or behavioral techniques — to become more rational and less disturbed and therefore better able to pursue their *own* goals for long-range pleasure and satisfaction. This usually involves helping them to pursue these goals within the context of their existing relationship (Ellis, 1957, 1978d, 1988b). However, in the course of counseling, it may become apparent that the long-range interests of both parties may be better served through separation or divorce. If so, your counseling may involve helping them dissolve their relationship with a minimum of emotional disturbance and pain (Ellis, 1978b; Ellis & Harper, 1961).

There are some distinct (and, we think, advantageous) differences between rational-emotive couples therapy and other approaches, such as systems theory, purely behavioral couples therapy, and traditional marital counseling.

First of all, most other approaches tend to give inadequate attention to the role of cognition in relationship difficulties. As Ellis (1978c, p. 42) points out, "disturbed marital and family relationships stem not so much from what happens among family members as from the perceptions that these members have and the views they take of these happenings." RET, therefore, encourages marital therapists to focus on cognitions, no matter what their theoretical orientation or treatment goal (Ellis, 1978c, 1978d).

Like family systems approaches, RET believes that a system is created by the way the individual members interact, but as Ellis (1986a, p. 4) has written:

> Focusing on wholeness, organization, and relationship among family members is important, but can be overdone. Families become disturbed not merely because of their organization and disorganization, but because of the serious personal problems of the family members.

Also, while RET focuses somewhat on creating environmental changes to ameliorate family problems (e.g., arranging for a nonassertive spouse to speak up), it particularly concentrates on creating attitudes that help family members feel less disturbed when unfortunate family conditions can*not* be changed.

RET acknowledges that disturbed interactions affect family members, but it holds that family systems approaches do not clearly specify the mechanisms whereby such systems develop and are maintained. RET proposes that the cognitions (and associated feelings and behaviors) of the individuals in the system lead to dysfunction, rather than the influences that somehow arise mysteriously from the system itself. Thus, people subject themselves to dysfunctional family patterns because they hold *beliefs* about events or anticipated rewards in the system. These beliefs often lead to disturbed emotions and reduced behavioral flexibility. Mental representation of the spouse and others *in the heads of* both partners largely *create* the "system" of unhealthfully interacting individuals.

Rational-emotive couples therapy includes considering the ripple effects that changes in one partner may have on other family members. In fact, using RET, you almost always investigate how a client's mate and other family members think, feel, and behave in response to the individual's changes. If irrational responses by close associates appear to be impeding the client's progress, you may attempt to work with the others in order to provide a more favorable interpersonal environment for the client's change efforts. You may encourage one client to use RET with the disturbed partner. And you may help the client to cope more effectively with others' irrational responses.

RET thus emphasizes the individual as well as the family and provides an answer to the fundamental question, "Who is the client?" that is different from that offered by other couples approaches — which tend to see the family, the system, or the relationship as the focal unit of study and intervention. RET assumes that *system* and *relationship* are words whose referents are really abstractions: properly used, they refer to patterns that observers and participants actively abstract, via their own cognitive processes, from ongoing interactions, and do not refer to some objective entity that is treatable per se. Instead of attempting to treat the abstraction as though it were an entity, with goals and interests of its own, you had better define *clients* as the individualss who come for help and then focus on helping them modify disturbed cognitions, affects, and behaviors that interact with those of their partners to create marital problems.

Emphasis on the individual as the focus of therapy also reflects RET's humanism (Ellis, 1962, 1973a; Walen, DiGiuseppe, & Wessler, 1980). Humanism places the highest value on the pursuit of people's personal happiness and sees relationships and social groups as valuable not so much for their own sakes as for their contribution to the happiness of individuals. Seeing the continuation of a marriage or relationship as an end in itself, or valuing it above the interests of the individuals involved, is inconsistent with humanistic philosophy.

RET does not give "communication" the special and rather sacred place that many marital therapists do. What may appear to be a communication skills deficit is often really an emotional problem on the part of the sender, the receiver, or both. People can beautifully send and receive their messages and yet make themselves furious when others do not comply with their "nice" communications. And people typically have cognitive schemas or "seives" to screen and interpret what they hear. While you may often train yourself to do active listening, you may be more concerned with correcting the systematic interpretive or evaluative distortions that your clients bring to the receiving and processing of their communications. Their irrational thinking and dysfunctional feelings and behaviors may well be your most appropriate therapeutic targets, for their "errors" in sending and receiving are often reflections of their emotional problems — especially anger — that you can track down to their cognitive instigation (e.g., shoulds, misattributions, damning).

RET also holds that total openness and honesty in communication is not necessarily to be highly valued, since it is often dysfunctional for a relationship. You may teach your clients to anticipate the likely consequences of their honestly speaking up, and to sometimes decide to refrain from shooting off their big mouths! Also, unresolvable issues and trivial matters that are not repeatedly communicated may easily contribute to a negative home climate. Likewise, bitching "communication" is not encouraged in RET. Rather, you may urge clients to make better choices, such as unresentful acceptance, active assertion, and consideration of unangry separation (see Hauck, 1981, 1984).

We believe that any kind of behavioral treatment, even the teaching of communication, social, or assertiveness skills, is often ineffective without examining the irrational cognitions that often block these skills. While it is very helpful to remedy real skill deficits, people usually engage in positive, helpful communication once their emotional blocks are minimized (Lange & Jakubowski, 1976; Wolfe, 1974, 1977; Wolfe & Fodor, 1975).

Chapter 5
Assessment Techniques

In this section we would like to discuss some initial interview strategies for rational-emotive (R-E) couples counseling. Most therapists working with couples tend to see the partners conjointly for the entirety of treatment. We believe this procedure is disadvantageous and recommend that one use a combination of individual and conjoint sessions for both assessment and treatment. For the initial session, it is often best to see both partners together. During this session, attempt to collect data about their agreed reasons for coming. Evaluate the nature and degree of *marital dissatisfaction* and what factors account for it.

Some important questions are: (1) Who initiated the request for counseling? (2) What is the nature of the disharmony? Too few rewards, too many costs? (3) Is the degree of marital upsetness equal in each partner? (4) Who gets upset at whom, how frequently, about what issues, and does what about it? (5) How do the partners solve problems? (6) How do they feel, think, and act when issues are unsolved?

This information is used to help you form a schema concerning the marriage. To acquire the information quickly, you require good interviewing skills. Few professionals are actually trained in marital, couples, or family therapy. Their experience may be limited to one course in their graduate education, supervision of a case or two during their internship, or some continuing education workshops primarily devoted to individual interventions. Some caveats may therefore be in order before you see couples.

First off, rational-emotive therapy (RET) is an active-directive therapy. Therefore, you usually get information by asking for it directly. DiGiuseppe (Whalen, DiGiuseppe, & Wessler, 1980) has discussed in detail why we believe that an active-directive approach to interviewing is helpful for building rapport and ensuring efficacy in therapy. Let us briefly underscore some of its essentials.

Therapists agree that rapport between therapist and client is helpful for ensuring effective treatment. However, in rational-emotive therapy, rapport is not deemed helpful or curative in, by, and of itself. Clients do not get better simply because of their good relationship with you. Rapport is helpful because, once it is established, clients are more likely to share their thoughts and feelings honestly with you. This helps you to achieve a valid and quick assessment of their problems. Also, rapport between you and your clients makes them more receptive to your educational and change efforts.

Rapport can be established in a number of ways. There are no exclusive techniques to develop it. Rapport is sometimes based on clients perceiving you as a sincere, honest, and understanding person. They infer these traits or attributes from many different behaviors which you may display. Reflection of feelings may be one such behavior, but it can also be inefficient for gathering information.

There are effective ways of establishing rapport which are also more efficient at gathering information. First, you can get right down to business. Clients come because they are in pain. They want to tell their story so that you can help them. You can best assure them by seeking specific information, explaining the purpose of your strategies, and offering techniques for helping couples to change their unhappiness.

Good questions designed to seek additional information about what the client has already told you show that you are listening. Developing hypotheses about the couple's relationship and their individual feelings shows concentration on their problems. Quickly suggesting rational cognitions and fulfilling behaviors reflects helpfulness. Testing your hypothesis by asking for feedback indicates collaboration.

Interviewing a couple is more difficult than is interviewing two clients singly. Partners' negativity, disruptive habits, and frequent arguments over details can easily distract you. We find that our interviews with couples elicit more information and fewer difficulties when we use the following guidelines.

GETTING BOTH SIDES

Often address your questions to one partner at a time. Questions that each partner can answer may create competition between the couple as to who will answer first or best. An old saying goes, "There are three sides to every story; his, hers, and the truth." When there is a particular issue about the relationship that you'd like answered, such as "How do they fight? Who takes charge of the children? Where and when did they get along best?" usually ask one mate first, and then also seek a second opinion from the other.

T: Rita, who do you think takes most responsibility for the children?
R: Well, I do except on weekends when Don takes over.
T: Don, is that the way you see it?
D: That's about it. I also take over on the evening when Rita attends school.

This style of questioning minimizes competition, acknowledges that each party may see things differently, and allows both partners to express their point of view. You can alternate who is asked questions first, so that the spouses feel they are equally participating in the process.

Try to spend fairly equal time discussing problems with both partners. This rule is the easiest to break when you focus on one member's disturbance. Thus, if John gets angry at Carol's spending habits, and she becomes angry and retaliates with more spending, you had better point out to both partners that their anger is hurting the relationship, that both can control their anger, and that both have their own idiosyncratic beliefs that make them angry. Then you can spend fairly equal time disputing the irrational Beliefs (iBs) of each partner. In this way, the responsibility for the disharmony is shared. Neither partner is blamed or scapegoated, and both are helped to overcome their beliefs which contribute to their disturbance.

However, if you deal only with John's anger at Carol's spending, Carol is left off the hook. This can be and often is interpreted by John as justification for his anger. You may thereby help reinforce John's irrational Belief that Carol absolutely must not overspend and is no good if she does. If the session ends before you get around to acknowledging Carol's role in the disharmony and disputing her own irrational Beliefs about getting back at John for his anger, more trouble may ensue. John may feel picked on and believe that you are taking sides. Carol may leave feeling vindicated and retaliate all week by more spending.

You may solve this problem by working with both partners in a structured fashion. First, you can reveal both partner's disturbed emotions. Second, you can show how each partner's upsetness keeps a cycle of disharmony and disturbance going, and you can indicate that you will give both time to work on their particular disordered feelings that contribute to the disharmony. Third, you can then spend some time identifying and disputing the irrational Beliefs that led to both spouse's disordered feelings and behaviors.

DEALING WITH DOMINATING PARTNERS

In many marriages, one spouse tends to dominate the other. In your joint sessions, the dominant member may speak for the more passive one. This presents a big obstacle for a valid assessment and effective therapy. For example,

> T: George, do you enjoy the social engagements that Jean plans with her sisters?
> J: Why, of course he does. George always has a marvelous time.

To prevent this disruptive interaction, try to pursue questioning until the partner answers for himself or herself.

> T: George, do you enjoy the social engagements that Jean plans with her sisters?
> J: Why, of course he does . . .
> T: I'd like George to answer for himself, Jean. Perhaps you could refrain from jumping in and answering for him. How about it, George? Do you enjoy them?
> G: Well, sometimes, but I don't like to go as often as we do.

Dominant spouses attempt to continue getting their way by hiding certain information, thereby making sure that the only opinions expressed are what they want presented. You may be an unwitting participant in this gambit by permitting the dominating spouse to answer for the other. By forcing both partners to answer questions directly for themselves, you invite the dominant spouse to change his or her controlling style. In addition, you may unearth problems not previously dealt with and teach the unassertive spouse new behaviors.

DID THE PARTNERS ANSWER YOUR QUESTION?

RET's explicit form of questioning is frequently new to clients, who are unfamiliar with its ideas and practices. Thus, they can easily confuse thoughts, feelings, and behaviors. You may ask a question designed to elicit information about thinking and your clients may respond in terms of their feelings and actions. Again, if you ask clients how they feel about losing a spouse, they may respond by telling you what a nerd the partner is. This tendency occurs more frequently with couples. Both parties have a number of gripes against the other, as well as various theories to explain the other's behavior. They frequently give you their hypotheses and attributions about their partner's acts instead of sharing their own irrational Beliefs and emotions about these acts.

> T: Jack, how do you feel when Shirley criticizes you in front of your friends?
>
> J: I feel she's trying to take out her anger toward her father on me. He always criticized her and she hates it. So I'm the scapegoat.

Note Jack didn't answer the question. He made no reference to his own emotional state. Rather, he provided an interesting hypothesis about Shirley's behavior. Here, it is wise to refocus the question back on the original topic, avoiding Jack's hypothesis or filing that away for later. If necessary, keep repeating the question until an answer is received.

> T: Jack, this might be true. But now I'm interested in your emotion. Let's focus on your feelings. What's going on inside your gut when she says these things?
>
> J: I feel she's a real bitch.
>
> T: Jack, you sound angry. And we can talk about that in a while. But, are you feeling only angry? What else are you feeling? Are you feeling sorry, hurt, or frustrated when she says these critical things?
>
> J: Well, more hurt than anything else. Well . . .

Your persistence may accomplish several goals. First, clients can learn to stop focusing on what the other partner does and focus on their own contributions to the marital problem. Second, they are encouraged to distinguish between facts, theories, opinions, and feelings. In addition, you discover what you want and can go on to other steps and procedures.

Couples who have been arguing for a long time frequently construct overgeneralized thinking. They describe their spouse as "always angry," or "she never speaks nicely to me," or "he never likes to do what I like." This "allness" thinking prevents them from compromising and achieving win-win positions. Their overgeneralizations are irrational ideas that lead to and enhance marital upsetness. You can helpfully ask questions that encourage specific complaints and goals, rather than those that solicit generalized "information." For example,

> T: Okay, George, what would you like to change that would give you more pleasure in the marriage?
>
> G: Well, we never get to do what I want to in our spare time. We always do what Jean wants.
>
> J: That's not true, George. How about all the time we visit the Smiths? We go because you like to visit, it's not my pleasure.
>
> T: Hold on, Jean. Let's try to pin this one down. What is it that you'd like to do for entertainment that you don't do now?
>
> G: Well, go to the movies more and play golf and maybe go out to visit friends.
>
> T: Okay, that's pretty specific. Can you think of anything else?
>
> G: No, not really.
>
> T: Jean, can you think of anything that George likes that the two of you could do but that you don't do very often?

J: No. Well, maybe what we could agree on watching TV. I guess I usually decide and George just goes along.

G: (Grunts)

T: Okay, George, now let's try to do two things. First, pin down some specific pleasures and how often you like to do them and, second, see what keeps you from doing them. Now, which activity would you like to talk about first?

Good assessment is a cornerstone of good treatment. Designing the treatment with no data is like writing in the dark. Traditionally, marriage counselors assess only the marital relationship. While it is important to get this information, it is incomplete. Much dissatisfaction and disturbance is instigated by private thoughts and feelings which are not always shared with one's spouse. For this reason, we recommend some individual sessions with each partner.

There are several advantages to individual sessions. The first and most important is determining each partner's agenda for seeking marital therapy. People come for couples counseling for many reasons, especially to help maintain and improve the relationship. However, many people who arrive at the marriage counselor's doorstep do not wish to continue with their present partner or are uncertain about doing so. Some clients have already half-decided to leave but are too frightened to do so because of fear of social disapproval or loneliness. They frequently engage in marital therapy to sabotage it. Or they hope that the failure of professional help may provide the needed excuse to separate. Alternatively, clients may differ about the type of relationship they want to build. One client may desire to have extramarital affairs on the side, and the other may vehemently oppose this. Some come seeking the aid of the therapist to get their spouse to bow to their own wishes. These are only a few of the many agendas you can discover and you will not properly address client goals if you are unaware of them.

Many clients who do desire to stay together have emotional concerns they are unwilling to share with their spouse. For example, they may be guilty about previous affairs or now desire to continue in such affairs. They may have extreme sex guilt which they are embarrassed to reveal to their partner. They may have intense anger at their spouse which they are not "supposed" to discuss. Consequently, many conjoint sessions may be needed before one partner becomes comfortable enough to talk about "shameful" topics. However, this information may be quite readily exposed and dealt with in separate individual sessions.

Sometimes the assessment discovered in individual sessions may help you determine the future course of treatment. You may then decide whether therapy had better continue conjointly or individually. You sometimes may see clients individually for a few sessions to help them deal with secret issues and then return to conjoint counseling.

You had better assess both clients' commitment to the marriage and their views of how it will foster their happiness. RETers do not insist on maintaining the marriage for the marriage's sake or because of social convention. But they do try to foster the personal happiness of both partners. So try to assess how rewarding the marriage is and how committed both partners are to it. One way to help clients estimate how happy they are in their marriage is to ask them if they have considered separation and, if not, to ask them to imagine how they would react to it.

This may be good strategy for several reasons. First, separation has usually crossed the partners' minds anyway, and it is diagnostic to get their thoughts on it. Some clients have decided that they desire a divorce and are coming to therapy to use it as an excuse to let the marriage fail. Such people may withhold this information because of their fears that you may oppose or disapprove of divorce. Or they may believe that you will not help them with antimarital feelings and decisions because you are a marriage counselor. By bringing up the issue and acknowledging that divorce is an alternative, you can communicate a noncondemning attitude toward it, as well as concern for the clients outside of their marriage. You can then discuss whether or not the partners want to separate, what the consequences of doing so may be, and what, if any, steps are to be taken to divorce.

Try to emphasize several important points when interviewing partners alone. First, the information discussed in the individual session is confidential and issues will not be discussed with the other partner unless the individual client desires it. Second, explain that most people have some secrets from their mates and it is this material that you would particularly like to discuss in the individual sessions. Third, don't push clients to act on any of the secret thoughts or desires privately discussed. You may sometimes encourage but not insist on more honesty with the partner. Fourth, to develop a plan to help the clients, you had better know as much as possible about their emotions and desires. Secret material is usually related to some emotional upset or else it wouldn't be secret. Fifth, try to determine the nature and extent of extramarital contacts of both parties. This information is helpful in determining their commitment to the marriage. Specific problems and clinical strategies to deal with problems revolving around infidelity will be discussed in Chapter 8.

Investigating the costs and benefits of separating helps clients make a full hedonic calculus in regard to their options. In marriage it is often easy to focus on the negative side of the relationship, and sometimes divorce and separation may seem to be a panacea. It's the "grass is always greener on the other side of the fence" syndrome. Conversely, being encouraged to imagine life without one's spouse may help point up some of the positive aspects which are often taken for granted. In addition, many clients fantasize about the advantages of a swinging single life but never think about it long enough to evaluate its negative aspects. Encouraging them to think about separation may help them focus on some of the cold realities of separating. The information revealed in obtaining ideas about separation may help you define the goals of both clients and determine if individual or conjoint sessions are most appropriate.

After the clients review the pros and cons of separation, several outcomes may emerge, such as these:

VARIABLE SATISFACTION WITH MARITAL UPSET

In many cases the cost-benefit ratio of the relationship is viewed as higher than other alternatives, even acknowledging some cost associated with marital dissatisfaction. For example, John and Mary get along well most of the time. The individual sessions reveal that John loves Mary very much, enjoys her company, and is committed to continuing with her. However, he experiences rage over the way she handles bank books, money, and the bills. His emotional upsetness tips the balance of a cost-benefit ratio in the unfavorable direction. John argues that if he could control his anger by accepting Mary's money problems, or if she could learn to be more orderly about finances, or if he took over the finances, the marriage would be workable. He is encouraged to think about pursuing one or all of these strategies.

At the same time, Mary is angry about John's anger at her. She finds this the worst thing about an otherwise fairly good relationship. John's rage tips her cost-benefit ratio against staying married. If John stops acting angrily, she would desire to stay in the relationship. One good therapeutic strategy would be to help both John and Mary *prefer* (but not *need*) to have the other's anger eliminated and *prefer* (but not *need*) the other's views about money to change. Then they could probably resolve their differences, make some compromises, and enjoy their marriage. Conjoint sessions are most likely to help them reach their desired goals.

Some clients may believe that the cost-benefit ratio is very poor for their marriage and wish to leave. They see separation as powerfully rewarding. However, they may be extremely fearful of the loneliness and the social stigma of divorce. Their anxiety and guilty tips the balance of the cost-benefit ratio toward staying. Such clients are in a classic approach-avoidance conflict. You can help relieve them by showing them how to reduce their anxiety and guilt and *then* decide what is better for them to do.

When clients believe that the cost-benefit ratio is against the relationship and have little or no emotional upsets, they will be most motivated to leave. Individual and/or conjoint sessions may be best geared to help them reassess their hedonic calculus and reach a decision. Some clients never really think through leaving. They fantasize and wonderfulize about it. When they realize there are many aspects of married life that they would miss, the rewards of leaving fade.

Once clients feel dissatisfied with an important aspect of marriage, they frequently engage in cognitive errors of selective awfulizing. When these errors are challenged, they frequently see their marriages are better than they first thought. Usually, the client who is least committed to the relationship has the most power. If both desire to stay, your best strategy may be to work first on the emotional problems of the least committed client, since that person is more likely to be the main force to break up the relationship.

Try to determine early in therapy to what extent irrational Beliefs are involved in a couple's difficulties. If they are *not*, and the problem is essentially one of dissatisfaction rather than disturbance, you can use cognitive questioning to help clients evaluate the pros and cons of their marriage. You can use behavioral interventions, such as contracting, to allow the couple to negotiate reductions in negative behaviors and increases in positive ones (Ellis & Harper, 1961; Stuart, 1980; Jacobson & Margolin, 1979).

The presence of irrational Beliefs can be elicited through direct questioning, through self-report inventories, or inferred from behavior. If a self-report questionnaire is desired, David Burns's (1984) BLAS test, which assesses the extent and "fit" of the marital partners' irrationalities, may be useful.

All the irrational beliefs that lead to individual disturbance may also create relationship disturbances. However, certain kinds of irrational beliefs seem to be particularly related to marriage. These include (1) dire needs for love and approval; (2) perfectionistic demands for self, mate, and the relationship; (3) a philosophy of blame and punishment; (4) beliefs that frustration and/or discomfort are horrible; and (5) beliefs that emotions *just* arise and are therefore uncontrollable (Ellis, 1982; Ellis & Harper, 1961).

Couples may, of course, develop their own idiosyncratic variations on these general irrational themes. For example, one couple may apply unrealistic standards and demands only to sexual behavior, another may apply them only to child-rearing practices, yet another may apply them to virtually every aspect of their relationship. Similarly, the dire need for love and approval may include beliefs that the individual, the spouse, or the relationship is worthless unless enormous affection is supplied. Discomfort anxiety—or low frustration tolerance (LFT), as we often call it in RET (Ellis, 1976c, 1979b, 1980a)—may additionally include other irrational Beliefs, thereby intensifying emotional disturbance.

You will want to be sensitive to "should" statements made by both clients, such as name-calling that suggests damning attitudes. Awful-izing will be indicated by extremist statements and low frustration tol-erance—"I can't stand it" philosophies. Irrational thinking patterns that are long standing, automatic, and unexamined are especially likely to interfere with a satisfying relationship. They crop up not only during an occasional fight, but over and over in the life of a relationship. You can find ample, repeated evidence that they exist.

You will want to observe patterns of communication to see if there are distortions in receiving or hostile tones in sending of messages. These may stem from emotional problems to be examined and treated by RET.

You will also want to assess any skill deficits, such as an assertiveness problem. Unassertiveness usually stems from underlying irrational thinking, such as, "If I speak up and tell my mate what I want and feel, I may get rejected and criticized, and that would be *awful* and would show how worthless I am!" (Lange & Jakubowski, 1976; Wolfe, 1974, 1977).

You can attempt to assess actual reinforcers provided by the partners to each other. Are they each satisfied with their sexual life? Are they respectful of each other? Is either partner being "paid off" in important ways that you had better know about (such as money and life-style advantages)?

What factors maintain problem behavior? What encourages couples to be "stuck" together in spite of serious disagreements and hassles?

Clients' ideas about rewards and the equity of their exchanges may have a powerful impact on their relationship satisfaction and, therefore, bear careful examination. Again, the basic ABC model (Ellis, 1973a, 1977a) and recent expansions thereof, such as the eight-step model by Wessler and Wessler (1980), provide a framework within which to ex-plore these cognitions. What are the partners attending to in their ex-changes, and how do they define and label what they perceive? What do they infer as to the probable causes, meaning, and consequences of a given exchange or exchange pattern? Having arrived at an interpre-tation of an event, how do they then evaluate what they think has happened? (Do they regard it as good? bad? indifferent? awful?) What evaluative criteria are they using, and are these preferences or absolutistic demands? Are clients attributing only bad motives to their spouses? Are they engaging in highly emotive styles of thinking (overgeneralized or black and white)?

Look at societal "myths" to which clients may strongly subscribe. Usually they will bring them up spontaneously in the form of aphorisms or personal laws. Ask about understandings clients had, when they first got together, about what they would give each other (what Sager, 1976, has called implicit marriage contracts). Discover what each partner expects of marriage and of the spouse, what "common wisdoms" they absorbed while they were growing up.

Family-of-origin *values*, incorporated early and without any reexamination during adult years, may form the basis for conflict today. Intolerant *belief systems* in several areas may lie behind conflictual relationships. What one mate *perceives* as a threat to his or her self-esteem may be the very thing that another spouse blindly *expects* that a "good" relationship entails.

Early cultural influences may have also shaped attitudes. Historical inquiry may help the partners see how their dysfunctional thinking came from family values, superstitions, and personal insecurities that are no longer relevant. Identifying their beliefs as continuations of childish attitudes may make it easier for some clients to give up their crooked thinking. However, if you are an RET therapist, you will not focus unduly on the roots of clients' disturbances, but rather on their active *perpetuation* of early irrational Beliefs.

Psychodynamically oriented family therapists are particularly interested in the ways that current family behaviors are transferred from early relationships. But it is likely that people disturb themselves through *reactions* to family teachings and that they *actively maintain* these early views and behaviors. Using RET, you may sometimes go back into clients' childhood experiences to learn about their patterns of thinking. But you need not do this routinely or in minute detail. You focus mainly on present disturbed thinking, even when it got its start many years before.

Look for distortions in the partners' perception of events experienced together—especially when what they tell you is very discrepant. Try to distinguish between neurotic distortions and more blatant psychotic processes.

Also, look for patterns of violence, substance abuse, habit problems, and irresponsibility that suggest the mates' very low frustration tolerance. By eliciting specific answers to questions about these issues, you discover the ABCs of a particular couple's exchanges and difficulties and help them develop an appropriate treatment plan.

Continue to assess the clients' problems as you proceed with treatment. Their responses to early treatment efforts often provide the most useful kind of diagnosis. Noncompliance with homework may suggest serious emotional blocks, such as anger and low frustration tolerance, that interfere with working on the relationship. You may also use "resistance" in therapy to make your assessment more specific, and you may combine cognitive detective work with functional behavior analysis to discover what rewards and benefits maintain the poor compliance in therapy as well as in the marriage.

Chapter 6
Treatment Techniques

Where both dissatisfaction and disturbance are involved in a relationship problem, rational-emotive therapy (RET) holds that the preferred therapeutic strategy is to work first on the *disturbance*. There are several reasons for this. First, it will often be extremely difficult to define clearly, identify, and reduce dissatisfaction until the overlay of disturbance has been ameliorated. Second, potentially helpful interventions against dissatisfaction problems are *un*likely to be maximally effective when one or both partners are emotionally upset. For example, it is difficult to get angry couples to comply with behavioral contracting procedures because they see little reason to try to please those with whom they are angry and little reason to stop engaging in behaviors designed to punish their "offensive" mates. Further, for they may often construe — or misconstrue — their mate's compliance with a contract as mere manipulative attempts to win over the therapist and get him or her to take sides. Initially, therefore, focus on eliciting and uprooting the irrational Beliefs (iBs) of both parties and attempt to resolve the disturbance before fully addressing the couple's dissatisfactions (Ellis, 1975b, 1982, 1986a).

You can also start with how the spouses may be disturbing themselves *about* their marital problems or about their decision to enter therapy. While these issues may be secondary to their main disturbances, until they are out of the way it is often harder to help the couple work on the primary issues. For example, the partners may believe that it is *awful* to have a troubled marriage and may therefore feel deeply ashamed to reveal marital problems, even to the therapist. Or, one of the partners may believe that people *should* always work out their own problems and may deeply resent the mate having made the therapy appointment. In both these cases you can question and dispute these irrational Beliefs.

You can also frame coming to therapy as a sign of health and hopefulness. The RET model shows people how they *can* change through conscious work and action. Couples do not have to wait passively for the partner to change or the marital situation to improve. RET helps people accept responsibility for their marital situation rather than accusing their mates of doing more damage to the marriage than they themselves.

As an RET practitioner, you often show how neither partner is in it alone nor lives in a vacuum. They *both* play a part in *both* the dissatisfaction and disturbance. Therefore, each partner is encouraged to bring up things about themselves on which they agree to work independently of (as well as with) their partner.

For a variety of reasons, clients often deny or resist accepting responsibility for their part in the relationship problems. Sometimes they are simply unaware of their contributions. They may have a distinct personality disorder (such as narcissism) or may have irrational Beliefs (e.g., "I am no good if I disrupt my marriage") that prohibit them from admission. These clients are the most likely to externalize the sources of their problems and enter therapy to help their partners change. Helping them admit to their negative roles is important in RET treatment.

Sometimes one partner takes the brunt of the responsibility for the marital problems. Since *one* person rarely is totally responsible and the other *totally* innocent, you can didactically and assertively explain the low probability of this occurring and show partners their responsibility for dissatisfaction and disturbance.

To engage resistant individuals to work on their part in the relationship disturbance, you can often show them how they are very powerful Activating Events (As) for their partners. Although they are not primarily causing their partners' craziness, they are usually responsible for *contributing* (as an "A") to it.

A	Activating Event–wife's *behavior* (e.g., continual complaining).
iB	husband's *irrational Belief* about her behavior (e.g., "She must not bitch so much! I can't stand it!").
iC	husband's *inappropriate Consequence* or *disturbance* (e.g., rage and depression).

If, in this case, you help the wife change the "A" which is presented to her husband, she will probably decrease their interactive difficulties. But, of course, you will also confront and discover the husband's irrational Beliefs about his wife's behavior.

The As (unpleasant Activating Events) that clients present to their partners are often their own Cs (emotional and behavioral Consequences).

A_1	unpleasant Activating Events experienced by wife.
B_1	wife's Beliefs about As.

C_1 wife's emotional and behavioral Consequences

B_2 husband's Beliefs about wife's Consequences.

C_2 husband's reactions or Consequences about wife's Consequences.

In working with couples, you point out this interactive framework in order to get both parties to accept at least part of the responsibility for the relationship disturbances.

Another problem that you often confront in couples counseling stems from what may be called "secondary Beliefs," that is, Beliefs that clients have *about their own* Consequences.

A_1 unpleasant Activating Events.

iB_1 irrational Beliefs about As.

iC_1 inappropriate emotional and behavioral Consequences of $A_1 \times B_1$.

A_2 Activating Events (same as C_1).

iB_2 irrational Beliefs about A_2.

iC_2 inappropriate emotional and behavioral Consequences of $A_2 \times B_2$.

As can be seen, the client's C can be an A not only for his or her partner but also for himself or herself. In relationship counseling, clients very often believe (at B_2) that their inappropriate emotions (iC_1) are functional, appropriate, and deserved. As a result, they do little to change this self-defeating Consequence.

The process through which clients learn that their negative emotions (at iC_1) are self- and relationship-defeating is called *functional disputing*. To help them perform a functional dispute, you challenge their beliefs regarding the functional nature of C_1. You commonly hear clients argue that "it is good to be angry" or "I have every right in the world to get mad." While it is true that they do have that right, is anger or aggression *helpful* in making their relationships better? Obviously not! Anger as a C for one partner is likely to activate the other's irrational Bs and lead to shared anger. As a result, the disturbance "rages" on!

Functional disputing, therefore, asks clients to explain or prove that their Cs are useful, productive, or helpful to their own and their relationship's happiness. When one partner asserts that "it doesn't hurt to be angry," you can immediately test this claim against the partner's perceptions. Usually, partners will argue that the other's extreme negative emotions are dysfunctional.

Even prior to working on marital disturbance, and prior to disputing functionally clients' beliefs about their Cs, you had better get agreement from both partners that they are committed to improving the relationship. That is, they accept the goals of increasing cooperation and rectifying their dissatisfactions. Once this commitment is secured, functional disputing can more easily proceed, for when clients commit to getting along with their mates, they can see that anger, for example, will not help achieve that goal.

Once a general commitment to get along is established, you can discover their individual goals and their commitment to work on them. Individuals can first generate their own goals. Later, their partners may add to this list. They can then learn how to challenge their irrational Beliefs to change their individual and conjoint disturbances.

When a client commits to make changes, the obvious question becomes: "What do I do to change?" Typically, clients believe that their emotions and behaviors directly stem from external Activating Events. If so, you show them how to make the B-C connection between Beliefs and disturbed Consequences.

Teaching clients the ABCs of RET shows them how to uproot the pernicious idea that disruptive emotions are externally caused and are therefore uncontrollable. Once they accept the idea that they themselves largely determine their emotional reactions, and see that they have a choice as to how they will feel and behave in response to any given Activating Event, they can then use the ABC model to challenge the various other irrational Beliefs that they may hold about themselves, their mates, and the relationship.

Teaching of the ABCs can be accomplished in conjoint sessions, with each partner learning from the therapist's work with him or her and the other partner. As you check for real understanding by clients that they themselves create much of their own disturbance, you can also show them that they can make themselves much less disturbed. This often produces a startlingly new perspective that is important in initiating the process of change.

Social psychologists point out that disputing social customs helps people to recognize that they actually live under "rules." Well-known family therapists like Milton Erickson and Salvatore Minuchin use this concept when they seek to upset customary family relationships to promote change. RET therapists also directly challenge clients and question their self-defeating assumptions. They do not subscribe to a nondirective, passive therapist role, nor are they neutral when it comes to dealing with clients' irrational and self-defeating ideas.

Using RET, you will tend to be direct rather than indirect (as are many family therapists). You will rarely try to "change" people without their awareness. Instead, you will attempt to educate them and make them consciously take charge of their own relationship — and, in fact, of their own lives. The major technique you can use to unsettle clients' "comfortable" malfunctioning is to dispute their irrational Beliefs.

Disputing involves any process where a client's irrational Beliefs and cognitive distortions are challenged and restructured. Therefore, you may be "technically eclectic" (A. A. Lazarus, 1981) in that you may employ any strategy that will help your clients restructure their faulty or crooked thinking. But you are not limited to strictly cognitive strategies and may employ a host of behavioral, emotive, imaginary, or interpersonal methods to accomplish this central goal. We will now discuss several types of disputational strategies that can be employed in couples counseling.

COGNITIVE METHODS OF RET

The most common disputational strategies are cognitive. That is, through discussion, you help clients to see that their irrational Beliefs are not empirically or logically based but are actually fallacious. You ask clients to prove or provide evidence to support their Beliefs. If they fail to provide evidence or you show them contradictory evidence, they often surrender their iBs. If evidence which supports the beliefs is uncovered, they are considered likely to be realistic or rational and are therefore not reconstructed.

Let us consider a typical irrational Belief that many of us have once held, such as the belief in the tooth fairy. Ask yourself this question: "Why do I *not* believe in the tooth fairy any longer? Why did I give up that idea?" Well, you most probably abandoned it because, upon further examination, you not only had no evidence to support the contention that a generous fairy entered your bedroom while you were sleeping to exchange your baby teeth for money, but you actually discovered evidence to contradict it. You learned that your parents actually made the exchange. You consequently no longer endorsed the childish fantasy.

Restructuring other iBs occurs in a similar way. And, as resistant as you were to giving up the tooth fairy, clients are equally resistant to changing their thinking. To dispute, you will ask them to prove their beliefs. Have them search for evidence bo prove or deny them. Do they make sense? Are they factually or realistically based? Are they rational?

You can also help clients to challenge the pragmatic nature of their iBs. You can ask them: "Is endorsement of that belief in your best interest?" "Does it help you to persist at thinking like that?" This is an important strategy since clients will often *choose* to hold on to the most irrational of beliefs because giving them up would be like losing an old and dear friend. It is hoped, and with effort, when clients see that a belief is false *and* is actually dysfunctional, they will then decide to work to give it up.

To use RET with couples, your major method is to expose and challenge irrational thinking, and especially that which is related to relationship disturbance. You may only discover few irrationalities–as when the couple is mainly rationally dissatisfied with each other, but also is doing some awfulizing about having problems and about possibly splitting up. Or you may find many irrationalities and have to decide where to start and on which beliefs to focus with which partner.

Disputing is a mainstay of RET treatment with couples as well as individuals. It can be done in conjoint sessions, but is sometimes more effective when conducted privately with one of the partners and then perhaps the other at a later time. Your style can vary from authoritative (not authoritarian), to persuasive, to humorous, to cajoling. One basic strategy is to ask unanswerable questions about clients' irrational Beliefs that point to their absurdity. They often respond as though a rational part of the belief has been challenged. You then show them what they have wrongly done and again try to get them to answer the question. Often, they cannot! For example:

T: *Why* must your husband stop drinking totally?
C: Because he's wrecking his health.
T: That's why it would certainly be better for him to stop, but you haven't told me why he absolutely must stop–why he really has no choice.
C: Well, it's a drag to live with him.
T: Yes, it certainly must be at times. But aren't you saying that because *you* want him to stop, he *must* do just as you say so that you can have it easier?
C: Well, I guess he doesn't *have to* do it just because I want it, but it would sure be better.
T: Yes, it would, and that's your sensible rational belief.

This example is a case where the therapist employs a Socratic dialogue to help the client to see that just because she wants her husband to behave in a certain way and thinks it would be better for the marriage (which may also be disputed), she does not need it that way. Her *preference* is not challenged, but her absolutist *demand* that her preference be satisfied is disputed.

Clients' irrational Beliefs may also be disputed by simply teaching the client what makes their thinking irrational and destructive. Didactic methods, using lecture, audiotape, videotape, or bibliotherapy can be very useful cognitive methods.

Other forms of disputing iBs include "*Where is it written* that you should have no frustration from your spouse?" "*Where is the evidence* that your husband is a rotten person?" When the clients respond, "I don't *want* frustration, and if my spouse gives me too much, I'll leave" or "My husband *acts* rottenly at times, and I'd better encourage him to change," they are shown how to strengthen these beliefs, which are rational alternatives to the demanding ones they also hold.

Another important way to challenge irrational Beliefs is to question their utility for clients' goals. This helps them to begin to rethink and restructure their dogmatic demands.

Of course, you will not dispute each and every irrational Belief that appears, but rather will want to select those that are typical of and basic to the marital disturbance. You can recognize such ideas by the frequency and degree with which they appear to underlie dysfunctional interactions. They will not usually be subtle or hidden. Your good assessment will repeatedly turn them up.

Commonly, a core irrationality consists of poor tolerance for that which doesn't come easily and comfortably. As I (A.E.) (1982) have noted, with amazing frequency, people in miserable marriages are affected with low frustration tolerance (LFT) — are first making themselves anxious, depressed, and hostile and are then drifting with their disturbed feelings about themselves and their mates and are doing little to take responsibility for them and to change them.

So you may spend considerable time on issues related to frustration tolerance. It leads to much anger over undesired partner behavior and troublesome marital events. Specifically, try to help clients to dispute the irrational beliefs associated with LFT (e.g., "I *must* not experience frustration or discomfort at any time, because that is *awful*! My spouse must *guarantee* that I do not feel uncomfortable or she or he is a *rotten person*!"). Helping clients to adopt a philosophy of long-term rather than short-term hedonism will aid them in reducing their LFT-related upsets. And it will enable them to achieve more long-range benefits by better tolerating the hassles they now define as "intolerable injustices."

As another major cognitive focus, teach your clients unconditional acceptance of themselves and others, since people-damning underlies so much disturbance in marriage. When partners are self-downing and consequently deny undesirable behavior, they often create dysfunctional interactions, and when they are judgmental toward a spouse, they will further worsen their problems. So encourage honest acknowledgment of poor behavior by both partners and help each to refrain from condemning the person who has shown the behavior. Nondamning of oneself and others is a powerful and helpful aspect of RET! (Ellis, 1957, 1962, 1972b, 1973a, 1976b; Ellis & Harper, 1975).

Several minutes of disputing irrational Beliefs, however persuasive you may be, are rarely enough to change prolonged habits or crooked thinking. So repeat your disputing many times and also use several other cognitive and noncognitive methods, as shown in the paragraphs that follow, to help modify these beliefs.

RET marital therapy utilizes many cognitive-behavioral techniques in addition to "preferential" RET, which strongly disputes clients' absolutist shoulds, musts, and commands. These include correcting faulty perceptions, inferences, and attributions; bringing partners' expectations more in line with reality; and providing them with helpful, rational things to say to themselves. These cognitive interventions test clients' perceptions of reality and ask whether what they see, infer, or expect match the real world. Therapists practicing Aaron Beck's (1976) type of cognitive therapy extensively use these methods of perceptual or empirical questioning but often ignore the musturbatory thinking that lies behind them and largely creates unrealistic views (e.g., see David Burns, 1980; Beck, 1988).

A useful way to rip up unrealistic perceptions is with the angry "attributions" that spouses often make about the "reasons" for the other's behavior. By helping clients to change such misattributions, you may well lead them to change their feelings and behavior. If a spouse interprets the partner's behavior as a personal attack, this partner may well become *angrier*. So you can question why this is the *only* possible explanation and try to get the client to generate other plausible explanations for the partner's "attack."

You may show a client that dubious attributions for a spouse's "bad" behavior may stem from this client's disturbance or from ignorance of what the other spouse wants or how to satisfy it. However, take care to make your reframings about the reasons for the spouse's behavior plausible. Also, do not push too hard against misattributions or argue with clients about their perceptions because this is less important than helping them think more rationally about situations whether they are correctly *or* incorrectly perceived. Thus, if clients say, "My spouse wants to leave the marriage," you may not argue with this misperception but may first respond, "Suppose she does leave, would that be disastrous? Could you not survive and still be happy?" Once they have made more rational appraisals of "worst possible cases," they do not tend to misperceive so many things as "bad" or "horrible."

You may direct cognitive restructuring efforts at faulty perceptions and inferences, if these indeed contribute to the couple's difficulties. Again, however, it should be noted that preferential or "elegant" RET differs from nonpreferential or "inelegant" RET—which Ellis (1980b) considers synonymous with general cognitive behavior therapy—in its strong, primary emphasis on helping clients revise their irrational evaluative cognitions, particularly their *shoulds* and *musts* that lead them to view various activating events as utterly *horrible* or *awful* instead of as relatively *unpleasant* or *bad* (Ellis, 1977a, 1978a, 1978c, 1979b, 1980a, 1982, 1985a, 1985b, 1987a).

Rational Coping Self-statements

Following the ABCs of RET comes Disputing D (as we have seen). Once irrational Beliefs are challenged, the Disputing person winds up with E, an Effective New Philosophy (that replaces unreasonable musts and commands with reasonable, alternative-providing preferences). Es can also be figured out by themselves and used by family clients to indoctrinate themselves with sensible coping statements (Ellis, 1973a, 1988a; Ellis & Abrahms, 1978; Ellis & Dryden, 1987; Meichenbaum, 1977).

Thus, you can help your couples to devise and repeat to themselves a number of rational self-statements, such as these:

"I don't *need* my mate to give me everything I want—although that would be nice!"

"Getting my partner to satisfy me sexually is *great* but not always *necessary*. I can also do a great deal *myself* to see that I am satisfied!"

"I very much *want* my mate to love me and pay great attention to me, but I can also be happy without these favors!"

"I greatly *desire* a lot of money and a beautiful home. But I am determined to live happily with my family even if we have much less!"

Psychoeducational Methods

As mentioned before, RET specializes in psychoeducational methods, because its goal is to reach as many people, including nonclients, as efficiently and intensively as possible. Although I (A.E.) devised RET for individual and group therapy in 1955, I saw a year later that it could be nicely put in book form and published my first book on it, *How to Live with a "Neurotic"* in 1957. This proved to be so successful, especially with married individuals, that I soon followed it with several other popular books, focused on individual as well as mating problems. These have included *Sex Without Guilt* (Ellis, 1958b), *The Art and Science of Love* (Ellis, 1960), *A Guide to Successful Marriage* (Ellis & Harper, 1961), the revised edition of *The American Sexual Tragedy*, (Ellis, 1954), *A New Guide to Rational Living* (Ellis & Harper, 1975), *A Guide to Personal Happiness* (Ellis & Becker, 1982), *How to Stubbornly Refuse to Make Yourself Miserable About Anything—Yes, Anything!* (Ellis, 1988a), and *Anger—How to Live with and Without It* (Ellis, 1977a).

You can follow the lead of the Institute for Rational-Emotive Therapy (IRET) in New York and give your clients a selection of RET pamphlets to read, as well as recommending some of the foregoing RET books. In addition, the IRET distributes many other good books and pamphlets that many couples find instructive — such as *Marriage Is a Loving Business* (Hauck, 1977), *Marital Myths* (A. A. Lazarus, 1985), *Male Sexuality* (Zilbergeld, 1978), *For Yourself* (Barbach, 1975), *Why Do I Think I Am Nothing Without a Man* (Russianoff, 1982), and *A Rational Counseling Primer* (Young, 1974).

For family members who particularly learn from audio and videocassettes, the IRET (45 East 65th Street, New York, NY 10021) distributes a number of items to which you may usefully refer your marital and family clients. These include *How to Be Happy Though Mated* (Ellis, 1975b), *Conquering Low Frustration Tolerance* (Ellis, 1972b), *Conquering the Dire Need for Love* (Ellis, 1977c), *Solving Emotional Problems* (Ellis, 1975c), and *Twenty-one Ways to Stop Worrying* (Ellis, 1973c).

The IRET in New York, as well as a number of other therapeutic organizations, each year gives a variety of talks and workshops, seminars, marathons, and intensives especially designed for married and would-be married people. Some of the recent events scheduled by the IRET include the following: Problems of Daily Living, Improving Social Skills, Romantic Love — Boon or Menace, Creative Encounters, Assertiveness Training, and Making Decisions and Solving Problems.

Cognitive Homework

RET almost always gives individual and marital clients regular cognitive homework, such as

Making a note of their disturbed feelings and behaviors during the week and discovering their self-statements (their iBs) that led to these dysfunctional Consequences (their Cs).

Figuring out and telling themselves several rational coping statements (rBs), particularly when they feel emotionally upset.

Figuring out other people's — especially family members' — irrational Beliefs when these others act disturbedly.

Actively disputing their own iBs.

Actively disputing — in their heads or in actual conversations–family members' and friends' iBs.

Filling out one or more RET Self-help Forms (Sichel & Ellis, 1984).

Semantic Methods

RET overlaps with the ideas of general semantics (Korzybski, 1933) and tries to help individuals and couples to make their language more precise, minimize their overgeneralizations, and thereby stop making themselves, as Korzybski nicely put it, unsane (Ellis, 1957, 1977a; Ellis & Harper, 1975). When, therefore, family members use imprecise, disturbance-creating ways of speaking, you can often correct them as follows:

If they say, "I *can't* get along with my mate," you help them change this to "I haven't gotten along with my mate yet, but there's probably no reason why I *can't.*"

If they say, "We *must* have a good marriage *at all times!*" you can help they say, instead, "We'd very much *prefer* to have a good marriage, but if we sometimes don't, we can live with our differences."

If they say, "My son disobeyed me and that *made me* furious," you can say, "You'd better change that to "My son disobeyed me and *I* chose to make myself furious."

If they say, "My in-laws keep interfering and I can't stand it!" help them change this to "My in-laws keep interfering and I keep *telling myself* that I can't stand it but I really *can*. I'll never *like* their interfering, but I *can* stand what I don't like!"

Other Cognitive Methods

RET uses a number of other cognitive methods in both individual and marital therapy, and material describing these methods is to be found in many articles and books, particularly those by Bard (1980, 1987); Bernard (1986), Bernard and Joyce (1984); Ellis (1962, 1971, 1973a, 1976a, 1979a, 1988a); Ellis and Abrahms (1978); Ellis and Becker (1982); Ellis & Bernard (1983, 1985); Ellis and Dryden (1987); Ellis, McInerny, DiGiuseppe, and Yeager (1988); Ellis and Whiteley (1979); Grieger (1988); Grieger and Boyd (1980); Grieger and Grieger (1982); Hauck (1980); McMullin (1986); Maultsby (1984); Walen, DiGiuseppe, and Wessler (1980); Wessler and Wessler (1980); and Wolfe and Brand (1977). These other cognitive techniques include cognitive distraction, persuasion, problem solving, goal selection, insight seeking, teaching self-acceptance, philosophic discussion, imaging, proselytizing, suggestion, modeling, listening to recordings of therapy sessions, sentence completion, self-

RET SELF-HELP FORM

Institute for Rational-Emotive Therapy
45 East 65th Street, New York, N.Y. 10021
(212) 535-0822

(A) ACTIVATING EVENTS, thoughts, or feelings that happened just before I felt emotionally disturbed or acted self-defeatingly: ————————————————————

(C) CONSEQUENCE or CONDITIONS — disturbed feeling or self-defeating behavior — that I produced and would like to change: ————————————————————

(B) BELIEFS — Irrational BELIEFS (IBs) leading to my CONSEQUENCE (emotional disturbance or self-defeating behavior). Circle all that apply to these ACTIVATING EVENTS (A).	(D) DISPUTES for each circled IRRATIONAL BELIEF. Examples: *"Why* MUST I do very well?" *"Where is it written that I am a BAD PERSON?" "Where is the evidence that I MUST be approved or accepted?"*	(E) EFFECTIVE RATIONAL BELIEFS (RBs) to replace my IRRATIONAL BELIEFS (IBs). *Examples: "I'd* PREFER *to do very well but I don't* HAVE TO." *"I am a* PERSON WHO *acted badly not a BAD PERSON." "There is no evidence that I* HAVE TO *be approved, though I would* LIKE *to be."*
1. I MUST do well or very well!	....	....
2. I am a BAD OR WORTHLESS PERSON when I act weakly or stupidly.	....	....
3. I MUST be approved or accepted by people I find important!	....	....
4. I NEED to be loved by someone who matters to me a lot!	....	....
5. I am a BAD, UNLOVABLE PERSON if I get rejected.	....	....
6. People MUST treat me fairly and give me what I NEED!	....	....

7. People MUST live up to my expectations or it is TERRIBLE!	....	....
	....	....
8. People who act immorally are undeserving, ROTTEN PEOPLE!	....	....
	....	....
9. I CAN'T STAND really bad things or very difficult people!	....	....
	....	....
10. My life MUST have few major hassles or troubles.	....	....
	....	....
11. It's AWFUL or HORRIBLE when major things don't go my way!	....	....
	....	....
12. I CAN'T STAND IT when life is really unfair!	....	....
	....	....
13. I NEED a good deal of immediate gratification and HAVE to feel miserable when I don't get it!	....	....
	....	....
Additional Irrational Beliefs:	....	....

(F) FEELINGS and BEHAVIORS I experienced after arriving at my EFFECTIVE RATIONAL BELIEFS: _____

I WILL WORK HARD TO REPEAT MY EFFECTIVE RATIONAL BELIEFS FORCEFULLY TO MYSELF ON MANY OCCASIONS SO THAT I CAN MAKE MYSELF LESS DISTURBED NOW AND ACT LESS SELF-DEFEATINGLY IN THE FUTURE.

Joyce Sichel, Ph.D. and Albert Ellis, Ph.D.   100 forms $10.00
Copyright © 1984 by the Institute for Rational-Emotive Therapy.   1000 forms $80.00

instructional training, stress innoculation, attribution retraining, corrective thinking, and so on.

These techniques are not just taught piecemeal or by rote, but within a general RET framework. This means that all family members are encouraged, if possible, to make a profound philosophical change, so that during and after therapy they fully accept grim realities that they can't change, give up nearly all absolutist, dogmatic thinking, and try to actualize themselves in more enjoyable ways.

EMOTIVE TECHNIQUES OF RET

RET uses many emotive methods of marital therapy in addition to reasoning and verbal persuasion because people do not usually change one irrational thought and then experience an immediate, profound major change in their feelings. Thinking, in its broadest sense, embodies emotions, and thought, feeling, and behavior profoundly interact (Ellis, 1962). People have "hot" thoughts as well as "cool" ones (Ellis, 1988a; Ellis & Dryden, 1987; R. Lazarus, 1982; Zajonc, 1980, 1984). They have impressionistic right-brain hemispheres as well as linear, logical left ones. So aim to engage people on their emotional level through a variety of techniques and to employ many rational-*emotive* techniques.

RET is far from emotionally flat. Even though you deal with reason, your therapy can be warm and concrete rather than cold and abstract. You can engage clients in deep and strong ways and be alive and vital with them. Here are some emotive techniques you can use.

Hypnosis

You can sometimes employ hypnosis, especially with those clients who greatly favor it and think that they can help themselves with it (Ellis, 1962, 1986b; Golden, Dowd, & Friedberg, 1987).

I (A.E.) have used hypnosis in recent years by putting people in a very light trance, telling them forcefully that they will discover their irrational Beliefs posthypnotically, will vigorously *Dispute* them, and will determinedly *act* against them. I make a recording of the hypnotic session, including the posthypnotic instructions, and have them listen to it at least once a day. By using this procedure, they often are motivated to work hard at RET and significantly help themselves (Ellis, 1986b).

Rational-Emotive Imagery

You can employ a technique called rational-emotive imagery (REI), developed by Maxie Maultsby (1975, 1984) and used in a more dramatic form by Ellis (1985a, 1988a; Ellis & Abrahms, 1978; Maultsby & Ellis, 1974).

Using the RET version of rational-emotive imagery, you can address your clients as follows:

"I want you both to use rational-emotive imagery regularly to help you change your inappropriate to more appropriate feelings. Let me show you, Diane, how to do this, and you, Henry, can also do it while I am working with Diane.

"Because, Diane, you said that you are often angry when Henry criticizes you, now I want you to imagine the worst possible thing in this respect. Vividly imagine that Henry keeps lambasting you for being so sloppy and untidy around the house. He really keeps sailing into you and keeps telling you what a slob and a rotten person you are. Can you vividly imagine his doing this?"

"I certainly can!"

"And how do you feel as you strongly imagine this? How do you honestly feel in your gut?"

"I think he's very unfair!"

"That's a thought, not a feeling. How do you *feel* as you're thinking that he's unfair?"

"Enraged! Homicidal!"

"Good. Really get in touch with that feeling. Let yourself feel very, very enraged."

"I do!"

"Good! Now, keep the same vivid image, don't change it, he's still lambasting you. Now *change* your feeling. Make yourself feel *only* appropriately sorry and disappointed—*only* sorry and disappointed—and not any longer angry."

"I'm not sure I can change my feeling."

"Yes, you can! Anyone can change his or her feelings—and so can you. You created your rage—now change it to *only* a feeling of sorriness and disappointment, *not* anger. Do it!"

"Okay. I only feel disappointed."

"Good! Now, *how* did you do it? What did you *do* to change your feeling?"

"I said to myself, 'That's Henry—that's *his* problem. Too bad—but I can take his unfair criticism and still be okay.'"

"Fine! That only took you a minute. Now what I want you to do every day, at least once a day, for the next 20 or 30 days, is to repeat what you have just done. Imagine the worst thing that can happen to you, such as Henry's steady and vile criticism. Let yourself feel, as you just did, enraged. Or depressed or panicked—or whatever inappropriate feeling you experience. Then change it to an appropriate feeling, such as sorriness and disappointment, the way you did, and other ways that will occur to you. Will you do this rational-emotive imagery exercise at least once a day, until you train yourself to automatically feel sorry and disappointed, instead of enraged, depressed, or panicked?"

"Yes, I will."

"Good! And if you don't, if you goof, you can reward yourself with something you find enjoyable only *after* you have done REI and changed your disturbed to appropriate feelings."

"I reward myself only *after* I have changed my inappropriate feeling?"

"Yes. And if you keep avoiding to do REI, you can also penalize yourself, by doing something unpleasant, every day you fail to do it."

"Like speaking to my mother-in-law for an hour? Would that be okay?"

"Fine! If you find that really penalizing, by all means use it. But one way or another, practice rational-emotive imagery until you really change your disturbed feelings to appropriate ones."

Evocative Imagery

You can use evocative imagery and have your clients imagine themselves thinking, feeling, and behaving in poor and in better marital interactions. Or you can use imagery for time projections into the future where better interactions are felt as possibilities. This kind of positive imagery is palliative, since it rarely helps people change their basic self-downing philosophies. But it can be temporarily effective.

Forceful Coping Self-statements

RET holds that, when they are disturbed, people *forcefully* and *vigorously* keep reindoctrinating themselves with irrational Beliefs and that really to give them up they had better *strongly* dispute them and vehemently replace them with more rational Beliefs (rBs) (Dryden, 1984; Ellis, 1985a, 1973b; Ellis & Becker, 1982). Thus, you can help couples and family members to say to themselves vehemently—yes, *vehemently*—coping statements like these:

"So my partner sometimes treats me unfairly! What partner doesn't! I'll not like it, but I definitely *can* stand it. Tough! But we can *still* have a good marriage!"

"I *want* to satisfy my mate sexually, and I shall keep trying until I do!" But I'm *not*, and *never* will be, a *total failure* if I don't! Just a fallible human who could be better at sex!"

"Raising my family is rough. But it's not *too* hard, and it *should* often be hard. No matter how hard it is, no matter *what* the hassles are, I *can* take it. And I *still* can enjoy family life!"

"I really don't *like* doing some things with my mate. And I don't *have* to! We can *both* enjoy different things and *still* have a good relationship! I have a *right* to be by myself at times, and if I am, I am *not* a *bad mate* or a rotten person!"

Roleplaying

As an RET practitioner, you can use roleplaying in marital situations, in several ways:

1. The partners may roleplay a typical argument, so that you can see how they fight and discover their irrational Beliefs and help them to dispute them.
2. You can let them roleplay an altercation, a communication problem, a difficult sex situation, or some other difficulty, show them a better way to enact this situation, and then have them practice the improved procedure.
3. You can let them roleplay, with yourself or each other, an anxiety-provoking situation—such as a job interview or talking to a stranger at a party. When they become anxious (or depressed or angry) during the roleplaying, stop the playing for a while to discover what they are telling themselves to upset themselves. Have them dispute their iBs at this point. Go back to the roleplay and show each one how to function better.
4. You can take the role of either partner and show a second partner how you would handle a difficult, argumentative, sensitive, or uncommunicative situation with the first partner. You can then reverse roles and indicate how you would act if you were the first partner.
5. You can take the role of an angry, anxious, or depressed family member, hold rigorously to this person's irrational Beliefs, strongly uphold these Beliefs (no matter how crazy they are), and get the disturbed family member to talk to you vigorously (playing himself or herself) out of these iBs.

Use of Tape Recordings

You can use tape recordings in several ways:

1. Encourage the partners to record each session with you and listen to the recording one or more times, to review the sessions—and hear them more objectively when they are not actually involved in them.
2. Encourage the family members to record some of their actual conversations with each other—especially their stiff arguments—and play them for you, so you can see what actually transpires at home, figure

out their irrationalities, and show them how to correct their defeating behaviors.

3. You can tape the sessions and from time to time play back parts of them to the partners, to show them what they actually said, the tone and manner in which they said it, and what they were telling themselves at these times.

4. You can get any or all of the family members who hold irrational Beliefs — such as "My mate should always do what I want!" — to state these on a cassette recording and then vigorously dispute them for three to five minutes. When they bring in these taped disputes, play them during the session to see how accurate and how *strong* their disputing is. Correct the content and power of their disputations and reassign this emotive homework again.

Use of Humor

RET holds that people had better take many things — especially their marriage — seriously but not *too* seriously. Emotional disturbance and marital conflict largely stem from *exaggerating* unfortunate events and their significance. As an RET practitioner, you can often use humor to show your clients how to see their marital and family problems in a less grim light (Ellis, 1977d, 1977e, 1987d; Fry & Salameh, 1987; Velten, 1987) and how to lighten their lives. Thus, you can

1. Humorously dispute both partner's irrational Beliefs and reduce them to absurdity.
2. Encourage the partners to look more humorously at each other's foibles and disruptive behaviors.
3. Assign family members to do some humorous shame-attacking exercises — such as walking a banana on a leash and feeding it with another banana.
4. Encourage overlyserious partners to do some humorous and playful things with each other — such as tickling each other or romping through the park with their children.
5. Show your clients that you can view some of your own mistakes humorously and not down yourself for them.
6. Show the couples you see how funny some of their behaviors are — as when they fight about sex and make themselves so mad that they withdraw from or have poor sex.
7. Teach your clients to take time out from their fights, silences, and emotional upsets by deliberately doing funny things, looking at humorous movies or listening to comedy routines, singing humorous

songs, reading comic material to each other, and engaging in other relaxing and interrupting humorous pursuits.

8. Provide your clients with some of the popular rational-humorous songs that they can sing to themselves or each other (Ellis, 1977d, 1977e, 1987d). Couples can especially use the following songs, sung to well-known tunes.

"WHINE, WHINE WHINE!"
(Tune, "Yale Whiffenpoof Song,"
by Guy Scull—a Harvard man!)
I cannot have all of my wishes filled—
Whine, whine, whine!
I cannot have every frustration stilled—
Whine, whine, whine!
Life really owes me the things that I miss,
Fate has to grant me eternal bliss!
And since I must settle for less than this—
Whine, whine, whine!

"PERFECT RATIONALITY"
(Tune, "Funiculi, Funicula,"
by Luigi Denza)
Some think the world must have a right direction,
And so do I! And so do I!
Some think that, with the slightest imperfection,
They can't get by—and so do I!
For I, I have to prove I'm superhuman,
And better far than people are!
To show I have miraculous acumen—
And always rate among the Great!
Perfect, perfect rationality
Is, of course, the only thing for me!
How can I ever think of being
If I must live fallibly?
Rationality must be a perfect thing for me!

"I'M JUST WILD ABOUT WORRY"
(Tune, "I'm Just Wild About Harry,"
by Eubie Blake)
Oh, I'm just wild about worry
And worry's wild about me!
We're quite a twosome to make life gruesome
And filled with anxiety!
Oh, worry's anguish I curry
And look for its guarantee!
Oh, I'm just wild about worry
And worry's wild about
Never mild about,
Most beguiled about me!

"YOU FOR ME AND ME FOR ME"
(Tune, "Tea for Two,"
by Vincent Youmans)

Picture you upon my knee,
Just you for me, and me for me!
And then you'll see
How happy I will be, dear!
Though you beseech me
You never will reach me —
For I am autistic
As any real mystic!
And only relate to
Myself with a great to-do, dear!
If you dare to try to care
You'll see my caring soon will wear,
For I can't pair and make our sharing fair!
If you want a family,
We'll both agree you'll baby me —
Then you'll see how happy I will be!

"I WISH I WERE NOT CRAZY!"
(Tune, "Dixie,"
by Dan Emmett)

Oh, I wish I were really put together —
Smooth and fine as patent leather!
Oh, how great to be rated innately sedate!
But I'm afraid that I was fated
To be rather aberrated —
Oh, how sad to be mad as my Mom and my Dad!
Oh, I wish I were not crazy! Hooray, hooray!
I wish my mind were less inclined
To be the kind that's hazy!
I could agree to really be less crazy.
But I, alas, am just too goddamned lazy!

"I'M DEPRESSED, DEPRESSED!"
(Tune, "The Band Played On,"
by Charles B. Ward)

When anything slightly goes wrong with my life,
I'm depressed, I'm depressed!
Whenever I'm stricken with chickenshit strife,
I feel most distressed!
When life isn't fated to be consecrated
I can't tolerate it at all!
When anything slightly goes wrong with my life,
I just bawl, bawl, bawl!

"LOVE ME, LOVE ME, ONLY ME!"
(Tune, "Yankee Doodle")

Love me, love me, only me
Or I'll die without you!

Make your love a guarantee,
So I can never doubt you!
Love me, love me totally—really, really try, dear.
But if you demand love, too,
I'll hate you till I die, dear!

Love me, love me all the time,
Thoroughly and wholly!
Life turns into slushy slime
'Less you love me solely!
Love me with great tenderness,
With no ifs or buts, dear.
If you love me somewhat less,
I'll have your goddamned guts, dear!
(Lyrics by Albert Ellis, copyright 1977–1988 by Institute for Rational-Emotive Therapy.)

In Vivo Emotional Techniques

Using RET, you may often help your clients to feel emotional during their sessions—not *merely* to get in touch with and express their feelings, but *also* to understand how they *created* them and *can change* them. Here, for example, are some RET in vivo emotional methods:

1. Encourage clients, by talk and exercises, to feel anxious, depressed, or angry during RET couples sessions. Thus, you can help them to fight with each other, to feel anxious about points you are raising, and to express their disappointment and depression about what is going on (or not going on) during the session. When their feeling is revealed, show them the rBs and iBs they are believing to largely create these feelings—and show them, right then and there, how to Dispute their iBs and change their inappropriate feelings.

2. Ask them, from time to time, about their feelings toward you and toward the therapy; determine whether these feelings are helpful or defeating; and show them what they can think and do to produce more of the former and less of the latter feelings.

3. Encourage them to get in touch with and express their feelings for each other (and for other family members), to be more honest about these feelings, to accept the consequences of having them, and to think and work at increasing some of them and decreasing others. Push them to feel and reveal their good and bad feelings in between sessions.

4. Urge them to practice feeling and expressing some of their held-in good feelings for each other during the sessions—and then to continue this expression during their regular marital lives.

5. Bring out their feelings for other family members (such as children and in-laws) during the sessions and help them tolerate their mate's feelings to which they object. Show them what they are probably telling themselves to create both their appropriate and inappropriate feelings and how they can think and act differently to minimize the latter.

Unconditional Acceptance

RET encourages you to use unconditional acceptance with all your individual and marital clients — to accept *them* as undamnable *people*, while often pointing out and showing them the ineffectiveness of the disturbed, foolish, and defeating *behaviors*. So work at — and, if necessary, get some rational-emotive therapy yourself — accepting and tolerating your clients — by what you say to them and by the tone and manner in which you say it.

RET, however, goes beyond Rogerian and other therapies in strongly *teaching* clients how to accept themselves, no matter *what* they do or fail to do. They can preferably do this by *only* rating or evaluating their *behaviors* and *not* their *selves, essences,* or *being*. But if they insist on giving themselves a global or total rating (as many of them will insist on doing), they can always *accept* themselves, or rate themselves as "good" persons just because (1) they are human, (2) they are alive, (3) they *choose* to accept themselves, or (4) they believe in an all-loving god or group that always loves them and gives them grace (Ellis, 1972c, 1976b, 1988a; Ellis & Becker, 1982; Ellis & Dryden, 1987; Ellis & Harper, 1975; Ellis & Whiteley, 1979; Ellis & Yeager, 1989).

Shame-Attacking Exercises

According to RET, shame (or self-downing, embarrassment, or feeling humiliated) is the essence of much human disturbance and often disrupts marital and family relations. Thus, because they feel ashamed, partners may not allow themselves to feel, may not express their feelings, may avoid various kinds of sex with each other, may refuse to accompany each other in certain activities, may resort to intense feelings and acts of jealousy, may not talk about many important issues, and so on. So, using RET, you can reveal couples' feelings of shame, show them with which irrational Beliefs they create these feelings, and teach them how to Dispute their iBs and surrender them.

Special RET shame-attacking exercises have been effectively used for many years (Ellis, 1969a, 1973b, 1988a; Ellis & Abrahms, 1978; Ellis & Becker, 1982; Ellis & Harper, 1975). You can use these with either or both marital partners in this way:

"Since you seem to be unduly ashamed of several things and needlessly put yourself down for doing them, or even thinking about them, I want you to experiment with some RET shame-attacking exercises. To do these exercises, you first think of something that you personally feel is shameful and something that you would particularly never do in public. Don't use anything that would harm yourself or get you in trouble — such as walking naked in public or telling your boss he or she is a louse. And don't harm anyone else — as by slapping them in the face or bothering them too much.

"Do something, instead, that you are ashamed to do because people would think you stupid or crazy and because you think you couldn't stand their disapproval. Like, for example, saying to a stranger. 'I just got out of the mental hospital. What month is this?' Or ask someone, 'Where is Fifth Avenue?' when you are standing on Fifth Avenue. Or get up at a lecture in front of a large audience and deliberately ask a stupid question. Or read a pornographic magazine in a subway train.

"Do two things while performing this shame-attacking exercise: (1) Do the acts you consider shameful in public. (2) work at *not* feeling ashamed or embarrassed while you are doing them.

"If you have trouble doing this exercise, you can reinforce yourself with something you really like only *after* you have done it and penalize yourself by doing something very unpleasant if you fail to do it."

BEHAVIORAL TECHNIQUES OF RET

The RET approach to marital treatment is highly behavioral as well as cognitive and emotive. Encouraging changes in clients' behavior is often an excellent way to get them to modify their ideas about what their relationship can be like and what possible roles they can play.

RET often incorporates George Kelly's (1955) idea that people are stuck in fixed roles but can break out of them by scripting new roles and trying them out experimentally. You can be a helpful guide in this process, encouraging clients to start behaving in new ways in their marriages — either ways that they have been afraid to behave (e.g., assertively) or ways they have been too angry to want to employ (e.g., believed they should not act lovingly to a poorly behaving spouse). These techniques may provide positive feedback to reinforce the new behavior and to modify dysfunctional beliefs about how spouses "must" behave in marriage. Behavioral techniques treat marital disturbance as well as dissatisfactions, so you can use them extensively.

When you treat dissatisfactions, you can approach a couple's problems with many behavioral techniques. Some are drawn from behavioral marital therapy because marital satisfaction increases when the partners can be helped to provide more reinforcements to each other. Also, contracting, negotiating, communication and assertiveness skills, and sex-

ual skills can increase the benefits coming to partners from their marriages (see, for example, Richard Stuart, 1980, on "Caring Days").
Other behavioral techniques include the following:

Skill Training

RET includes skill training, especially sexual and social training and interpersonal training (Ellis, 1958b, 1960, 1969a, 1976a, 1979a, 1988a; Ellis & Becker, 1982; Ellis & Conway, 1967, Ellis & Harper, 1961, 1975). You can show your marriage and family clients how to acquire skills in assertion, in communication, in family planning, in money management, in sexual relating, in making friends, and in other important areas where any of the family members (or all of them) are deficient. Naturally, using RET you try to discover what your couples clients are telling themselves to block their acquiring important individual and social skills. But as you help them to change their blocking irrationalities, you may often show them how to acquire and keep practicing useful family and life skills.

Bearing Frustration

Low frustration tolerance may well ruin more marriages than any other human trait—since marriage and family life *is* frustrating, and when partners have great LFT, they procrastinate, avoid responsibilities, take their mates for granted, dress and keep house slovenly, neglect their children, keep losing jobs, and let a hundred other important family obligations slide. They also often gamble, heavily drink, smoke, overeat, and indulge in other obnoxious habits (Ellis, 1973a, 1979b, 1980a, 1985a, 1988a, 1988b; Ellis & Becker, 1982; Ellis & Dryden, 1987; Ellis & Whiteley, 1979).

You can often show couples what drivel they are telling themselves to create and perpetuate the LFT—such as "It's *too* hard to do things when my mate wants them done. It *shouldn't* be that hard! How awful! Screw it—I won't do it!" Helping clients to see that marriage often *should* be hard and that it's *not* awful to assume its responsibilities undercuts their LFT and often improves their marriage.

One behavioral method of helping clients to ameliorate their LFT is to encourage them to stay in *un*comfortable situations until they become comfortable (and sometimes enjoyable) and until they reap suitable rewards from doing so. Thus, you can help your family clients

To stay in "rotten" marriages until they really work at improving them—or discover that they are unimprovable.

To keep being unangry and kind to difficult family members until these individuals become less difficult.

To talk intimately to each other until they feel comfortable doing so.

To try "unpleasant" or "disgusting" sex acts their partners desire until they become comfortable with them or until they find they are not really worth the trouble.

To tolerate "boring" social affairs until they lose their anxieties about engaging in them.

To stop smoking against their mate's objections until they become comfortable not smoking.

To assume family responsibilities and stop defining them as "too hard" or "awful."

Reinforcements and Penalties

As noted throughout this book, RET frequently uses reinforcements to help people do difficult tasks, and it is famous for its encouraging people to enact penalties — such as burning a hundred dollar bill — when they fail to carry out important assignments (Ellis, 1969b, 1988a; Ellis & Becker, 1982; Ellis & Dryden, 1987; Ellis & Whiteley, 1979). Using RET, you can encourage couples to reward or reinforce themselves *after* they have done promised acts, such as:

Remembered their mate's and children's birthdays.

Saved certain amounts of money.

Taken the trouble to satisfy their partner sexually.

Shown regular signs of verbal and nonverbal affection.

Been nice to their in-laws.

Refrained from yelling at their children.

Taken their mate out to dinner.

Invited friends to their home.

Talked to their mates at mealtime.

Planned a family outing.

Helped clean the house.

Shopped for food.

By the same token, if either of the mates promises to do something, such as the things just listed, and fails to carry out his or her promises, this mate can take on stiff penalties such as:

Burning a hundred dollar bill.

Eating some obnoxious food.

Talking to a boring person for an hour.

Cleaning the toilet.

Fixing the house.

Babysitting.

Watching a type of movie he or she hates.

Getting up an hour earlier than usual.

Driving the car for several hours.

Attending a disliked social function.

In Vivo Desensitization Homework

RET favors active, in vivo desensitization homework assignments to help clients overcome their anxiety, depression, rage, compulsions, obsessions, phobias, and other neurotic problems (Ellis, 1957, 1962, 1971, 1976a, 1977a, 1979a; Ellis & Becker, 1982; Ellis & Grieger, 1977, 1986; Ellis & Harper, 1975; Ellis & Whiteley, 1979; Grieger & Boyd, 1981; Walen, DiGiuseppe, & Wessler, 1980; Wessler & Wessler, 1980; Young, 1984). You can give your marital and family clients various activity assignments and can at times try to help them do these implosively—that is, many times in quick succession—instead of more gradually. For example;

They can experiment with sex acts that they are neurotically avoiding.

They can stop arguing after ten minutes.

They can spend a half hour a day talking about their feelings.

They can plan and carry out pleasurable activities.

They can do shame-attacking exercises.

They can engage in new family functions.

They can divide up and perform various household chores.

Assertiveness Training

You may often employ assertiveness training. Fear of asking for better treatment often reflects a client's dire need for love. People may fear that assertive requests will prompt their partner to stop loving them, or even to leave them. Because they believe that this would be catastrophic, they tolerate exploitative behavior by their mates rather than risk losing them.

In such cases, you can empirically dispute the fearful partner's inference that their mate will reject them or leave if they behave assertively. However, this may be an inferior strategy because it leaves the client's underlying musts, shoulds, and absolutist needs intact. Almost all spouses will get angry or annoyed at some point if assertively asked to do something they consider inconvenient or unpleasant, and some may actually withdraw their affection or leave. Even if this is unlikely, it is certainly possible, and an empirical strategy leaves the client ill-prepared to cope if disapproval for assertiveness does occur. Your preferred strategy, therefore, is to work for an elegant solution, challenging the clients' belief that they desperately need love and that it would be catastrophic to lose it. Once this is accomplished, you can help clients more calmly evaluate the probability that assertive requests will lead to rejection and encourage them to seek greater equity in the relationship (Ellis, 1979a; Wolfe, 1974, 1977; Wolfe & Fodor, 1975).

Partners who feel guilty or ashamed about asking for more equitable treatment often are chronic self-downers. People with serious self-rating problems often believe that they are totally unworthy and undeserving of good treatment. They consequently tend to believe that unfair treatment by their spouse is appropriate, that it would be inappropriate and shameful to ask for more consideration, and that doing so would therefore make them even wormier than they already believe themselves to be. In other words, chronic self-downers paradoxically manage to perceive unfair treatment as fair, given their own low opinion of themselves. You often had better use intensive individual RET to combat their self-downing problems before such individuals can begin to assertively negotiate for improved equity and satisfaction in their relationships.

Use of Logical Consequences

People not only define equity differently, but they may also differ substantially in their beliefs and expectations about it. Their beliefs may be either rational or irrational. Using RET, you can predict that people who adhere rationally to a strong desire for equity in their relationships will feel appropriately dissatisfied, disappointed, or annoyed when real inequities occur and will accordingly make active and constructive attempts to improve matters. Others, however, may go beyond preferring equity and tack on irrational, absolutistic demands that they be treated fairly. When clients with such beliefs encounter inconsiderate situations, as they almost inevitably will, rational-emotive theory predicts that they will feel disturbed and behave dysfunctionally. You therefore had better not only address clients' views of equitable exchange, but also their demands and expectations about equity.

Using RET, you will be interested in teaching the partners how to relinquish their demands, yet try to shape each other's behavior by using rewards and penalties (à la B. F. Skinner) so that they feel more satisfied with what they are getting from their mate. Paul Hauck (1984) has adopted many Adlerian ideas about consequences to show spouses how they can unangrily "protest" bad behavior in their partner by staging sit-down strikes and being otherwise uncooperative until their *wishes* are met better.

Charles Huber (Huber & Baruth, 1989) has also written from an Adlerian perspective on incorporating the work of Rudolf Dreikurs into RET therapy, helping a spouse devise and enforce "logical consequences" when there are not "natural consequences" for poor behavior on the mate's part (for example, not having dinner ready for a mate who repeatedly comes home from work very late without calling). We suspect that these techniques are effective not only because the errant spouse learns that "there is no free dinner," but also because the victimized spouse has an appropriate outlet for rational or appropriate displeasure.

Problem Solving and Use of Hedonic Calculus

You can also draw on two major behavioral techniques that help clients to approach life in a rational manner. They are *rational problem solving* and *the hedonic calculus*. While you can use these techniques with your individual clients, they are especially well suited to marital concerns. Rational problem solving is a well-known behavioral approach (see, for example, Spivack, Platt, & Shure, 1976) and has been applied more directly to RET by Harold Greenwald (1981) in direct decision therapy.

To use problem solving, show marital clients that they have more than one alternative action and that they can take a more active approach to solving their practical problems. When partners are depressed, the use of this method is likely to help them restructure some of the beliefs that make them depressed—for example, that they are stuck, helpless, and hopeless in the face of a bad situation.

You can also frequently help the partners use a hedonic calculus. This involves having each spouse weigh (from their own point of view) the costs and benefits of alternate courses of action—for example, whether to remain in a relationship or to leave it. Where the partners have already been thinking of leaving, it helps them bring personal taste and common sense to their decision, and where they had not openly considered it, they can feel immense relief in exploring their options. If you work with spouses on weighing the advantages and disadvantages of their marital decisions, you can also better assess their thinking disturbances. You can pinpoint emotional blocks to taking certain actions that did not emerge earlier in assessment.

Reframing

RET has always used the cognitive method of reframing clients' "bad" or destructive beliefs and putting them in a favorable, constructive light. Thus, if a couple views their arguments as "terrible" and "unbearable," you can sometimes show them that these arguments may in some ways be defeating but that they may also indicate healthy assertion and self-expression and may, if continued in an unangry way, lead to a resolution of some of their conflicts. If one partner complains that the other is rarely companionable, you may show the deprived mate that he or she has plenty of time and space to grow and develop and to seek out enjoyable private pursuits. If both partners are frustrated by conventional sex, you can point out the advantages and the adventures of experimenting with unconventional outlets (Ellis, 1988a; Ellis & Becker, 1982).

RET offers family members another, somewhat special kind of reframing. As Ellis (1973b, 1984b, 1988a, 1988b) has noted for many years, users of RET can take up the gauntlet and accept the challenge of stubbornly refusing to make themselves miserable about anything. Thus, you can show your clients that even if they have a very bad or incompatible marriage, even if one of them is physically handicapped, even if one mate dies many years before the other, even if a couple very much wants children but is permanently childless—in all these unfortunate situations, and many more, you can challenge your clients to feel appropriately sad, sorry, and frustrated, but *not* severely anxious, depressed, or hostile. By using RET—including many techniques outlined in this chapter—they can reframe their practical and emotional problems as intriguing and fascinating difficulties to be solved rather than as "holy horrors."

Referenting

When you try to help marital or family members with compulsions (e.g., incessant talking), with addictions (e.g., alcohol and overeating), with severe avoidances (e.g., proscrastination), or with phobias (e.g., sex phobias), you may use referenting to encourage them to stop an obnoxious behavior (Danysh, 1974; Ellis & Harper, 1975). With referenting, they write down a list of the disadvantages of indulging in the undesired behavior (e.g., smoking, drinking, or overeating) and a list of the advantages of *not* engaging in this activity. They then review these lists several times a day to remind them of the value of giving up their compulsions and phobic avoidances. You can check their agreed-upon referenting, to see that they regularly do it.

OTHER THERAPY METHODS

Overcoming Resistance

You can deal with "resistance"to change in RET marital treatment in much the same way that you deal with other emotional problems in the couple's life—by looking for irrational Beliefs and reinforcers that are maintaining self-defeating behaviors. The beliefs may include neediness, perfectionism, and demandingness.

Irrational Beliefs are often mediators or "reinforcers" for antimarital behavior. Certain "benefits" are highly reinforcing because of the *receiver's* irrational thinking about them. For example, "My wife does everything for me, and I couldn't possibly give that up because it would be *awful* to have to take care of my own life!" And "If I change, my husband will feel very threatened and may not stick by me like he does now. I *need* him to stick close by me—I need it more than anything in the world! I can't do *anything* to jeopardize his staying!"

Wherever possible, concentrate on challenging those irrational Beliefs that create disturbed emotions and poor marital behaviors. This helps spouses successfully change their strategies and either raise their marital satisfaction or prepare to part less stressfully. Note again it is usually best to try to enhance both partners' happiness—whether within the marriage or without. Specific methods of overcoming resistance to change by using RET are covered in detail in Ellis (1985a).

Interpersonal Strategies

Useful interpersonal strategies involve one partner helping the other partner change his or her thinking, and vice versa. It is important, however, to first work for a reasonable degree of *cooperation* between partners and a *commitment* to work *constructively* before teaching them how to do interpersonal therapy. Otherwise, clients may sabotage their partner's progress to prove how crazy or uncommitted he or she really is.

1. *10 Rounds*. This strategy parallels what occurs in a boxing match. In a typical match, fighters fight for three minutes per round with one minute between rounds to regroup and receive coaching from their corners as to how to win the fight. This is typical of couples' confrontations. Between "rounds" and punches, partners often coach themselves as to how to better hurt their mates. Often, too, they don't even take breaks between rounds. You can recommend to couples that they are allowed to fight but had better do so in rounds where the one-minute rests are used to remind themselves to use constructive rather than destructive interventions. Also, they are to be coached (by themselves) in their corners so as to increase rational thinking and minimize the disruptive emotions that will likely exacerbate their fighting.

2. *Up Front Reminders No. I*. Assuming a *commitment* to work together *cooperatively* and *constructively*, "up front reminders" can help couples "turn off" their disturbing disagreements.

Couples are generally very aware of the slings and arrows that they throw at each other during times of confrontation or disagreement. A list of these "daggers" can be made during a therapy session, with both partners agreeing that these are detrimental to the relationship and that they commit to stop doing them. Each partner then agrees to say, *when one of these obnoxious acts is occurring*, "I would like you to stop this behavior" and the other will agree to stop it. Each partner, therefore, acts as a cue person to help the other cease and desist. He or she can show the partner their contractual agreement where their "daggers'" are listed and where a commitment to change is signed. If either partner refuses to cooperate and change his or her behavior *on the spot*, these events will serve as grist for the next therapy session.

3. *Up Front Reminders No. II*. When clients are in cooperative modes of thinking, we recommend that they make a list of their true attitudes regarding their partners. For example, one attitude might be: "Even though I sometimes yell at you, it's just because I get myself crazy. Don't think that I don't love you, because I do." When one partner is acting "crazy," the other preferably should remind himself or herself of

these previously articulated messages so as to prevent himself or herself from falling victim to the spouse's "craziness." This will also remind the "crazy" spouse of the agreement both made to *stop* their relationship-defeating behaviors.

4. *Partner as Therapist.* When one partner behaves disturbedly, the other partner can act as an RET therapist and help change his or her thinking so as to relieve the unnecessary emotional distress. When the partner or therapists do this, they will automatically be reminding themselves to be aware of their own crooked thinking.

5. *Reinforcement Times.* You can encourage clients to sit each other down and commend each other on any successes they've had managing their disturbed emotions. They can also go over the situations where they were not particularly successful and try to discern *constructively* the irrationalities that made them disturbed. For both situations, the partners work with each other to assess crooked thinking patterns while at the same time reinforcing *cooperation* of their mutual attempts to rectify their problems and doing preventive work for future problems.

6. *Other Interpersonal Strategies.* There are many other creative interpersonal, cooperative, and constructive strategies in which couples can be engaged to help them overcome their relationship disturbances and dissatisfactions. You can use your ingenuity to create, modify, and tailor specific exercises to your particular clients.

Chapter 7
RET Approach to Sexual Problems

It has been said that the most important sex organ is between the ears, and RET's cognitive-behavioral approach to sexual problems confirms and applies this view. It emphasizes that *knowledge* and *attitudes* about the body, sexuality, sexual performance, and sexual problems importantly affect the kind of sexual adjustment people will make. Therefore, RET's primary approach to sexual problems is cognitive — focusing on client's crooked thinking to reduce dysfunctional emotions (like anxiety) and to enhance enjoyment. RET also employs many *behavioral* methods to reduce sex anxiety, improve skills, and modify sabotaging sexual attitudes.

I (A.E.) have been a sex therapist even before there was a recognized specialty in the field. In early publications (1954, 1958b, 1960), I suggested that guilty and shameful thoughts were a major block to sexual enjoyment. While social and familial disapproval of sex has lessened, you may still find much sexual guilt, puritanism, and shame among your clients — and if so I would recommend that their self-downing thoughts be assessed and dealt with early in treatment. Then they can unanxiously focus on their other sex problems.

Emphatically dispute any self-downing ideas about body, performance inadequacy, or "dirtiness." You may also find self-denigration by people who do not have very exciting sexual lives. Even if their performance is adequate, they may "should" on themselves about having *too* mild sexual enjoyment and refuse to berate themselves however they perform (Ellis, 1975a, 1976a, 1978c, 1980c, 1980d, 1988a).

You may find that women with orgasm difficulty are increasingly hard on themselves now that the society has developed a new myth that all women are potentially multiorgasmic. So encourage the nonorgasmic woman to accept herself as a person who may not have great

77

explosive sex but is in no way an inferior person. Hold out hope that she may be able to get more sexual enjoyment in the future, but show her that she can still have quite a happy life without great orgasms.

Low frustration tolerance (LFT) is seen in many clients, especially those who are greatly upset about having sex problems. They often believe that they *cannot stand* their particular problem or that it is really *too difficult* to overcome. They are impatient for treatment to work—demanding that things *must* be solved very quickly. Dispute these ideas vigorously and show clients that whining will do little to alleviate their distress—that, in fact, it creates anxiety about anxiety and exacerbates their basic problems (Ellis, 1979b, 1980a).

Clients are looking for magic pills that do not exist in the real world of sex. They had better change their attitudes and *work hard* at changing what they are dissatisfied with. It they are not willing to work at changing themselves and helping their spouse, they had better gracefully accept the situation as it is (or decide to leave their sexual relationship).

Among some male clients, machismo is still very much present. You may find men who demand studlike sex performance from themselves, as well as reassuring admiration from their partners. They have over-bought the kind of societal myths we discussed in the first chapter. These clients may feel distress over minor performance problems—such as occasional erection difficulties or lack of desire—especially as they go through their middle years. They are highly anxious or depressed because they connect hypermasculinity with worthiness. As an RET therapist, you can educate these clients about normal sexuality—strongly correct their unrealistic expectations. But you can focus even more on disputing their irrational thinking about the dire necessity for phenomenal sexual performance, and you can vigorously challenge the awfulizing and self-downing that these clients attach to less than stud-quality intercourse (Ellis, 1980d).

Some clients are not anxious about their own performance but are angry at their partner's sexual behavior. They have rigid standards for their mates to follow. You can teach tolerance and actively dispute the idea that one's partner *must* exactly fulfill one's sex preferences.

Often one partner wants sex more frequently than the other, or wants a broader range of sexual activities, and goes on to demand that the spouse comply. Try to help such clients see that adults don't have to always get what they want and that a satisfying compromise may well be achieved—as they give up their demandingness and their consequent emotional disturbance.

Another way in which anger worsens sexual problems is when non-sexual anger is expressed in the sexual area. Sex may be withheld or certain acts forced on a partner. You can help clients to feel displeased instead of angry and to stop using any avenue (including the bedroom) to discharge rage. Many sexual difficulties also reflect a relationship problem. When individuals are disturbed within their marriage, they are also likely to be less functional in their bedroom.

You can distinguish between *sexual dysfunction* and *sexually related disturbance*—a distinction similar to that you can make between *marital dissatisfaction* and *marital disturbance*. Behavioral techniques are often useful for sex dissatisfactions as well as for dysfunctions. You can offer clients many behavioral techniques to help with their problems of sexual functioning (e.g., using sensate focus to aid copulation and the squeeze technique for premature ejaculation). However, it is often wise to delay using these techniques while you first work on their emotional disturbance. Try for "elegant" acceptance by the clients of themselves and of their partner—even if their sex problem cannot be substantially improved. Keep the sexual problems in a general perspective. And try to avoid awfulizing to yourself about clients' sexual dysfunction.

When you see clients with substantial sexual *dysfunction,* such as primary lack of orgasm, unconsummated marriages, and vaginismus, you may well have them see a medical doctor as you proceed. Assuming there is no underlying organic problem, attempt to restructure unhelpful attitudes and give behavioral assignments (such as the sensate focus on a couple for whom sex has become adversive or masturbatory exercises for nonorgasmic women).

You can also supply accurate sexual information to modify unrealistic attitudes and strategies. Use models, diagrams, and helpful books, such as Zilbergeld's (1978) one on male sexuality. For women, you may recommend books on orgasmic training, such as Barbach's (1975). Even in this enlightened time, there are still many sexual misconceptions that color the way a couple approaches sexual life. So not only dispute their irrational Beliefs, but also help them to obtain more accurate information. An RET therapist, Susan Walen (1985; Walen & Bass, 1986) has noted people had better be aware of cognitive components of sexual matters like arousal, to decide whether to let arousal continue or not.

Clients may also avoid sex practices that were unacceptable when they were young (e.g., oral techniques). Male clients may benefit from instructions about what women often desire in sex (e.g., tenderness, cuddling, direct oral or manual stimulation of the clitoris). When they then do not act to satisfy their mates better, you may suspect that they are angry or have low frustration tolerance.

It is often a relief for men to hear that they do not have to rely only on their sacred penis to satisfy their partner. I (A.E.) am sometimes especially blunt with clients who refuse to see beyond intercourse as a way of having mutual sexual pleasure. This is usually highly therapeutic for men who suffer from anxiety about erections. Many couples continue to hold the highly limiting idea, however, that all sex must consist of intercourse or else it is second rate. So they remain hung up on penile-vaginal copulation (Ellis, 1976a, 1977b, 1980d).

Once sex failure has occurred, partners may awfulize or damn themselves about it. This will lead to anxiety about the future and depressed feelings about the past. They may focus unduly on doing well in sex to *prove* rather than *enjoy* themselves. When they become critical spectators of their own performances, they deaden sexual response. To be an effective RET therapist, short-circuit your clients' leap from devaluing their performances to devaluing their *selves*. You thereby encourage them to have less compulsive spectatoring and less obsessive focus on sex performance (Ellis, 1976a, 1980d; Ellis & Harper, 1975).

When men fail sexually, they *and* their women often blame themselves—especially for having bodies which they perceive as insufficiently attractive. You can therefore correct inaccurate attributions that such spouses make about their sexual problems. You may sometimes encourage the spouses to share their negative perceptions and inferences, so that misunderstandings can be corrected.

In case of a male's chronic failure, assess the extent to which the problem seems to have been created and sustained by anxiety. When anxiety exists, use RET to help reduce men's sacredizing sexual "success." Dispute catastrophizing thoughts ("I'll *never* satisfy a woman!"), and stress the client's ability to have an adequate sex life even without intercourse. Once a man is able to be more relaxed *about* his problem, the problem itself tends to be much less frequent. If you encourage a man to focus on enjoying himself in ways that do not depend on an erect penis, he not only commonly enjoys himself more but also is able to experience adequate erections. Often probe for the irrational thinking that ties poor sexual performance to low self-worth.

There is a very useful paper in the spring 1986 edition of the *Journal of Rational-Emotive Therapy* by Susan Walen and Barry Bass on the treatment of specific sexual problems with RET. On the importance of providing accurate information, the authors provide some excellent examples of a fifty-year-old woman who "had for years been rubbing a hemorrhoid, not her clitoris" and other women who expect that if they are able to have an orgasm that it will be "a Hollywood-style fit, complete with skyrockets and sonic booms rather than a spiral reflex. Occasionally such a woman will discover that she'd been having orgasms all along, only she didn't recognize them for what they were."

You can show some clients that thinking *unsexy thoughts* interferes with their having a sexy time. Unsexy thoughts include "I *must* please my partner!" "It's terrible that I'm frustrating my partner!" "I mustn't take so long (or so short)!" "My partner *should* do more for *me*! He's a rotten bastard!" Help your clients be more casual and less grim about perfect sexual performance. In a reciprocal relationship, each person will at times be more satisfied than the other, and that can be fine as long as it is not always one-sided, or if there is nonsexual compensation for ongoing sexual disappointment.

You may encourage your clients to face honestly whether they are a good sexual partner for the other. Often, one partner's insensitive or defensive avoidance prevents him or her from being more satisfying to the other. Mates never have to berate themselves if they haven't been doing a good job, but you can strongly encourage positive behavior change in the interests of the marriage.

As an RET therapist who tends to be tolerant about sexual matters, you can encourage clients to engage in beneficial behaviors about which they may feel ashamed. Improvement under these circumstances is often very rapid. For example, a spouse who has been masturbating to satisfy sexual desires in between marital sexual sessions may feel guilty and uneasy about this "solution," yet it may be a good one. Or a spouse who engages in homosexual fantasy during married sex may be reassured (usually in a private session) that it is not uncommon, not criminal, and also does not need to be acted upon outside the marriage. You can encourage your clients to change what can be changed—regardless of how long poor sex has continued—but to accept what is probably not going to change. To accept something does not mean you have to like it.

At times you can do assertiveness training with clients—usually wives—who have not made known what they really want sexually from their partners. This can distinctly facilitate marital *satisfaction*, of course, and it can also lessen marital *disturbance*. When you do assertiveness training, look for any irrational thinking that has blocked your clients from being more assertive. Look for rigid ideas about "what nice girls do and don't do" and beliefs about the awfulness of looking awkward or of being disapproved for having "wrong" sexual desires. Women may particularly shy away from asking for manual or oral stimulation of their clitoral region because they believe this is shameful or would be an *awful* burden for a partner. You may want to ask women clients specifically whether they are getting the kind of stimulation from their partner that allows them to be as orgasmic as they can be through masturbation. Women who are sexually unsatisfied may be both self-hating and angry at their partner who has not "read their mind" better. Their men may know only vaguely that something is wrong or may feel confused or guilty or helpless concerning the woman's lack of pleasure. Both partners may be caught in a syndrome of faked orgasms which relieve some emotional pressure, but which generate other poor results.

You may sometimes treat cases where there is an unusual sexual preference — either for abstinence or for some sex practice that is preferred by one partner but not the other. You can then encourage both partners to be less demanding about performing or avoiding this practice. Once they are calmer, if is often possible for them to speak up assertively for themselves and to negotiate a compromise. Sometimes partners can agree that preferences which they do not share will be satisfied outside the marriage, although fear of sexually transmitted diseases has reduced the feasibility of this strategy.

Recently, extramarital sex has probably diminished because of realistic concern about disease. Making a satisfactory sex life *within* the marriage is becoming more and more important to couples, and marital therapists are being called upon more frequently. However, there is still much interest in extramarital sex, and it is important for you, as an RET marital therapist, to convey a nonjudgmental attitude toward extracurricular sex, while scrutinizing the clients' reasons for wanting it. As I (A.E.) wrote in *The Civilized Couple's Guide to Extramarital Adventure* (Ellis, 1972a), which the world found rather shocking, extramarital sex can be chosen wisely or unwisely and can be practiced in a discreet, civilized, *or* highly damaging way. Disturbed reasons for seeking outside partners include low frustration tolerance for working on marriage problems, hostility toward one's spouse, and undue need for ego bolstering. Challenging the irrational Beliefs of errant partners may help them make wiser decisions about their sexual lives within and without the marriage.

Transcripts of therapist-client dialogues showing how sex problems are handled in the case of RET sessions are presented in several books, including Chapters 10 and 11 of *A Guide to Successful Marriage* (Ellis & Harper, 1961), Chapters 2 and 6 of *Growth Through Reason* (Ellis, 1971), and Chapter 10 of *A Guide to Personal Happiness* (Ellis & Becker, 1982). An excerpt from the case of a couple with a sex problem follows:

Husband: We're both very dissatisfied with our sex life. It's practically nonexistent. She's never interested.

Wife: What do you mean "never"? You just want to do it and that's it. Whatever happened to our feelings during sex? You're right, I'm really not interested in wham, bam, thank you Ma'am!

Husband: Don't start that shit, Miss "Holier than Thou."

Wife: What "shit"? You *don't* treat me like a woman when we make love. Actually, we *don't* make love. We make sex.

Husband: Maybe if you were a little more like a woman, you'd get treated like one. Instead, it has to be just right. Conditions have to be perfect.

Wife: That's right. Otherwise, you could just go to some "professional" to be serviced.
Husband: Serviced? Well, you just lie there. What do you expect?
Wife: Love. Caring. Tenderness. Feelings. [pause] Affection. [pause] *Not* horseplay.
Therapist: Let's hold up for a second here. Can I assume that you want to improve your sex life?
Wife: Yes, of course. But . . .
Husband: [cutting her off] I don't know if we can. It's been a bore.
Wife: Then go outside of our marriage for it.
Husband: Maybe I should.
Therapist: [cutting them both off] You both seem to get pretty upset over this problem. [to husband] How do you feel about the problem?
Husband: Like it is her fault. She should just loosen up . . .
Therapist: Those are your *thoughts* about this situation. But how do you feel?
Husband: Pissed off.
Therapist: [to wife] And you?
Wife: I get angry and depressed. I just can't take this any more. He should be more sensitive. I'm not that experienced. What does he expect?
Therapist: So you both *feel* angry.
Husband: Absolutely.
Wife: Yes, most of the time.
Therapist: What role does your anger play in terms of helping you get beyond your problem?
Husband: [more calmly] Well . . . I admit that it probably only distances us more.
Therapist: Probably?
Husband: Definitely . . . but I personally can't help it. How would you feel if your wife rejected you?
Therapist: I understand it's hard, and you admit that it interferes with your getting over the problem.
Husband: Sure.
Therapist: [to wife] What are your thoughts about the role of anger in this situation?
Wife: I think it's a function of frustration. Both frustration with each other and pent-up sexual energy.
Therapist: How might anger reduction facilitate the sex therapy process, then?
Wife: I think we'd work better together. Or at least we would be more willing to try to work it out more.
Husband: Yeah. At this point, we don't ever rationally try. I think we both probably just turn each other off even more with our respective anger.
Therapist: Then let's take a look at your respective anger.

[NOTE: The couple presents a great deal of information up to this point in the session. We can start to hypothesize that they possess very different ideas about sex. The husband appears to be less romantic and the wife appears more traditional. However, had the therapist immediately explored their individual attitudes about sex and what sex *should* be like, he or she would likely have met their respective anger as an obstacle. The therapist, then, focuses the therapy toward reduction of their individual disturbances about their sexual dissatisfaction.]

Therapist: What do you [to both] see as the source of your anger toward each other?

Husband: Her attitudes about sex.

Wife: His whole manner . . . about sex.

Therapist: Okay. You are both offering that the source, or cause, of your anger is your partner's attitudes or behaviors. In other words [to husband], she makes you and and [to wife] he makes you angry.

Husband: Yes.

Wife: Yes.

Therapist: How does this happen?

Wife: Well, he gives me "that look" or . . .

Therapist: [interrupts]. No. I'm not asking *what* he does. I'm asking *how* does he, or for that matter how *can* he or anyone *make you* angry?

Wife: I'm not sure I understand.

Therapist: You are both saying that something outside of yourself actually *causes* anger in you. Is that what you mean?

Husband: Yes, absolutely.

Therapist: Let's look at this somewhat differently for a moment. Can either of you conceive of a different emotional response, other than anger, to your spouse's behavior?

Wife: Sure.

Husband: What do you mean?

Wife: She means, we could get depressed or even fearful rather than always angry. Right?

Therapist: That's right. Isn't it true that you do, in fact, experience different emotions in response to your spouse?

Husband: Yeah. Sometimes I don't care. Other times I get really angry.

Therapist: Well then, if your partner's behavior and your sex problems cause your anger, how do we explain or account for depression, apathy, fear, and any other responses?

Wife: Sometimes I don't think about it.

Husband: I sometimes make it more or less important, depending upon the moment.

Therapist: So you are both saying that your particular emotional response is a function of *how* you are thinking about the problem.

Wife: I see.

Husband: That's right. But what are we supposed to do . . . try to *like* what we really don't like?

Therapist: No! That would be *rationalizing* or bull-shitting yourself. What we want you to do in order to minimize your negative, inappropriate and extreme anger is change your attitude in a more realistic or rational, not rationalizing, direction.

Husband: I really get myself pretty irrational and crazy.

Wife: I think we both forget our general attitude, which in the past has always been constructive. Now we are pretty much just destructive. I think we probably both really distort things and get ourselves nuts.

Therapist: So the *source* of your respective anger is . . .

Wife: Ourselves.

Husband: Our crazy ways of thinking about our problems.

Wife: But my beliefs about sex don't seem crazy to me.

Therapist: Even a person's most irrational and self-defeating beliefs don't *always* seem crazy to them. We all often fail to detect or identify our irrationalities. However, rather than talking about your beliefs that cause or contribute to your sex problem, we did agree to focus on managing your individual and collective anger which is a function or product of your thinking. Let's look at your individual thoughts or beliefs about your spouse and your problems which make you so angry. Remember, you agree that you both want to reduce or eliminate your anger.

[NOTE: The therapist establishes the relationship between thoughts and feelings and is ready to assess and dispute the beliefs which cause their anger.]

Husband: Okay.

Wife: [nods] All right.

Therapist: Think about this for a second. What are your *thoughts* about your partner's behaviors that make you so angry? What goes through your head about this problem? In other words, what do you *tell yourself* about it?

Husband: That she should be more open . . . more interested and receptive.

Therapist: When you say "she should," what do you mean?

Husband: She should be more active, you know.

Therapist: I'm sorry. I still don't know what you mean when you say she *should* be more open, active, and so on.

Husband: I mean that it would make our relationship better and our sex life better.

Therapist: That's likely. But you are answering a different question from the one I asked. I asked: "What do you mean 'she should' take a different approach to sex?" But, you answered the question: "Why might it be better or preferable?" Tell me, why *should* she act differently? Just becuase you'd like it?

Husband: Because that's how good marriages work.

Therapist: Well, that's probably arguable, but, for now, I'll accept that point of view as valid. However, even though it would be preferable and even though it might increase the likelihood of helping out your relationship, why *must* she act differently?

Husband: She doesn't *have to*! Obviously. But I'd surely like her to.

Therapist: It's really not so obvious. Right now you probably realize that she does *have to* act according to the way you'd like her to act. But this does not mean that you won't continue to want her to change her sexual ways. But, when you are getting yourself really angry, are you telling yourself and irrationally demanding that she *must* act differently, or are you more realistically and rationally saying that you'd like a change but it does not have to be?

Husband: I'm demanding.

Therapist: Which results in what?

Husband: Only anger and, as we said before, turns both of us off to each other. [to wife] I'm sorry. I'm going to work to get myself less crazy and demanding.

Wife: I guess I am pretty demanding, too.

Therapist: How's that?

Wife: I think that I pretty much demand that he take on my attitudes about sex and what it should be like.

Therapist: That's interesting. You both share, essentially, the same irrational belief, namely, "sex *should be, has to be* my way."

Husband: I admit that. But I don't agree that wanting it to be different is all that bad.

Wife: Neither do I. And although we agree that we both *irrationally* demand it our way, we still have a conflict. We *want* it in different ways. What do we do with that?

Therapist: Well, up this point, you haven't really cooperated with each other in working out this conflict. Right?

Husband: Right!

Wife: Mmm-hmm.

Therapist: The obstacle to cooperate being . . .

Wife: Anger. It pretty much poisoned us. It became *de*structive.

Husband: Yeah! I refused to even consider her feelings. It had to be my way. *No* compromising! *No* negotiations!

Therapist: I'm glad to hear that you are acknowledging what the source of your *disturbed* conflict is — your demandingness and anger.

Wife: We have to manage ourselves first so we'll have a shot at working this whole thing out.

Therapist: That's right. Now that you are both somewhat less disturbed and angry with each other, and you seem to be more cooperation-oriented, let's take a look at your beliefs about sex which led to your conflicts. Why don't each of you try to identify your individual demands or rigid doctrines about what sex is supposed to be like.

Husband: I've always believed that the wife should be available for the husband when he wants her. I see sex as wild and passionate. That's what I believe it is supposed to be like.

Therapist: Supposed to be like?

Husband: You know what I mean.

Therapist: No, I don't.

Husband: Well, not *supposed* to, I guess. But that's how I'd rather it be.

Therapist: Which is it? Does sex *have* to be active, wild, etcetera? Does it *have* to be the way you *want* it to be?

Husband: Well . . . no.
Therapist: You don't sound convincing.
Husband: [stronger] No. It doesn't have to be my way. But I would rather it be *more* of my way, at least sometimes.
Therapist: That sounds more reasonable. [to wife] What do you think?
Wife: I prefer it to be soft and romantic. It should be more love than just sex. And the time has to be right.
Therapist: It sounds like you have almost diametrically opposite demands or requirements about what sex or love-making is supposed to be like.
Wife: I guess these *are* demands, aren't they?
Therapist: Yes. Now, why does sex *have* to be love-making? *And,* why do you *need* perfect conditions?
Wife: Because that's what makes it love! That's what I see it as involving.
Therapist: I understand your preferences. But, you are saying that you *must* have it the way you *prefer* it to be. Why does it *have* to be the way you want it?
Wife: It doesn't have to be my way all the time. But I would like it that way more often.
Therapist: So, you don't need it to be a certain way.
Wife: No.
Therapist: [to husband] Do you?
Husband: No.
Therapist: So neither of you really *has to* have it your way. What does that mean?
Husband: That I can lighten up my expectations, or should I say, requirements. And try to be more affectionate.
Therapist: [nods]
Wife: And I feel more willing to "free up" a little, but it will probably take some time and patience.
Husband: Be patient with me, too, okay?
Wife: [agrees]
Therapist: [smiles] You seem to be interested in cooperating and negotiating with each other on this. Is this the same two people I met earlier? What happened?
Husband: Well, for me, I realize that I was acting like a spoiled child, needing things *my* way or no way. Actually, I believed I *needed* it my way. No one cooperates with a childish belief like that.
Wife: I guess we shared the same nutty demand. It just appeared different on the surface. If I remind myself that we don't *have to* do it my way, I'll probably relax and be more spontaneous. That is what he wants.

[NOTE: The therapist then gave them a homework assignment to remind themselves and each other at prescribed periods during the day that they *do not* need things their own way. They were also given RET homework sheets to dispute their self-defeating have-tos both in acute situations and prophylactically.]

Chapter 8
RET Approach to Jealousy

Jealousy is a common problem in marital relationships. The extremely jealous mate is likely to be a very unhappy, insecure person and to make the partner's life much more difficult, too. Jealousy is often not itself a simple emotion. It usually includes intense anxiety and obsessive thinking, as well as intense anger (with a potential for violence). Jealous individuals are also highly subject to depressive states.

We can conceive of jealousy as a "cognitive-affective constellation" since it is comprised of both thinking and feeling processes. Strong jealousy involves irrational thinking. Possessive people *evaluate* retaining the loved person as essential to their status, security, and happiness. They think they must *own* their partners. As Paul Hauck, an RET therapist, has written in a useful self-help book on jealousy (1981): "Even if she makes love with her old flame right in front of you, that won't make you jealous unless you let it. Granted, it is not proper behavior for a wife. And for you to disapprove of it and be saddened by it would be perfectly normal. However, to become filled with rage and want to kill someone is neurotic. And you are the only one who can do that to yourself."

"Rational" jealousy involves thoughts about wanting to keep one's lover, to avoid sharing one's time with him or her, and to perceive oneself as less entitled when closeness is disrupted. Potential loss is evaluated negatively and leads to much sadness—but not to fury or despair (Ellis, 1972a, 1984a).

Fury and despair are the jealous responses to *irrational thinking*, such as "I need my spouse desperately, and it would be the worst thing in the world to lose him or her; I am nothing without him or her; he or she must stick by me; it would be the cruelest act in the world for him or her to abandon me." As a result of these ways of thinking, the highly jealous person keeps scanning the environment for signs that the spouse may not be perfectly faithful. Infidelity is readily imagined; antennas are expected to spot it, since it represents such an extreme danger to the jealous person. Naturally, this leads also to paranoid investigative behavior, to attempts to restrict the spouse's activities, and to ugly scenes confronting the spouse with his or her supposed misdeeds.

Jealous clients exhibit childish commandingness. While they protest enormous, undying love for the mate, they can also become so angry that the mate is declared better dead than bedded with another love. They are dogmatically convinced that if the lover has violated a "contract" for inordinate love and exclusive attention, he or she is a totally bad person who deserves to be punished by the little prince or princess for failing to be a good subject (Ellis, 1972a, 1984a).

No wonder this pattern leads so often to marital problems! While the spouses of a very jealous person may initially be flattered, they soon feel harassed and resentful—especially when they have to restrict their lives to please their paranoid spouse. Life becomes bent to the jealous one's irrational needs. It is like living with a tyrant.

Using RET, you will go after the delusional component of pathological jealousy. But you will mostly dispute the core irrational beliefs that create possession anxiety and insecurity.

Don't merely reassure your clients that abandonment will surely not occur. You have no way of knowing that for sure—and no one can give guarantees about the future. Even if the spouse is obviously faithful, clients who get used to reassurance will keep seeking it whenever a new occasion for doubt arises. They never learn to undisturb themselves, or to face the future, whatever it holds, without terror.

So look for the *core* beliefs underlying jealous insecurity. These beliefs tend to be rather primitive ones about the self and one's safety in the world. Very possessive people may literally believe that they are less than a whole person (and really in danger) without a special companion or caretaker. (This lack of root identity is especially prevalent in borderline personalities.) Try to expose and dispute their highly irrational thinking and also use emotionally evocative methods to uproot their strongly held ideas.

Jealous people frequently have what I (A.E.) have called "the dire need for love" (Ellis, 1957, 1979a, 1984a, 1984b, 1988a; Ellis & Harper, 1961, 1975). They experience this need like a highly dependent infant, when, in fact, they can be helped to see that they are adults who will not wither without care.

Try to determine how jealous clients *think* when their spouse engages in some trigger activity, and show that their irrational Beliefs lead to their disturbed emotions and behaviors. Teach them the ABCs of RET and help them realize that it is not their spouse's *actions* that gets them disturbed, but their own highly demanding, catastrophe-predicting *thinking.* Show them how their catastrophizing repeats itself across situations and leads to the same obsessive pattern.

Aim for the "elegant" solution so that clients view the possible loss of their lover as an *unfortunate* but hardly a *horrible* event. Model the attitude, "If it happens, it happens—I might be temporarily knocked for a loop, but I will cope with it, and I certainly won't have to be destroyed by it." Also, help them separate abandonment from self-worth and future lovability. "Even if my mate wants another person, it doesn't prove that *I* am rotten and unlovable!"

Severe anxiety and depression are usually paramount with jealous people. But also reveal and dispute their irrational Beliefs that generate intense anger, since anger is frequently prominent. Anger-producing thoughts are typically beliefs such as "You, my partner, *must* help me to feel secure because absolute trust is so important to me. How rotten you are if you make me insecure!" "You *must* need me as much as I need you, or you're a miserable, ungrateful bastard!" Help clients to see the illogic of these grandiose demands and dispute actively their own demandingness.

Especially where unfaithfulness has actually occurred, try to dispute the ideas that underlie the European-like idea of the "cuckold": "My mate had *no right* to put me into this position!" You may help the cheated-upon one to attribute the spouse's behavior to the partner's *own* desires rather than to demeaning intent. But also go on to dispute the idea that anyone else can truly *lower* a spouse. Jealous people *give* their mates "power" over them. While it is likely that the relatives and neighbors will see them as fools if their spouse is unfaithful, they could live with it even if some did. You can show them that it is hardly the worst thing in the world if infidelity occurs (Ellis, 1972a, 1984a).

Besides cognitive work with a jealous client, you can also use *behavioral* assignments. These may include acting lovingly but *not* overpossessively. You can coach some jealous clients in assertive skills where their spouse seems to have been taking advantage of them. More important, you assign the jealous clients, no matter how they feel, to refuse to *display* jealousy. Convince them that they can control their behavior, even when they are anxious and when behaving in a new way seems unnatural. Point out to them and have them make a list of the damaging effects wrought by their actions, and help them force themselves not to indulge in obnoxious old behaviors (frequently checking up on the spouse, "testing" them, badgering and quizzing, etc.).

You can often be quite blunt with jealous people. Show them that if they go on as they have, they will in fact create the situation they fear the most—their spouse will become so disgusted with their jealous, tyrannical behavior that he or she will probably leave. Focus on the long-term costs of relieving their anxieties by checking up on or limiting the spouse's freedom.

You can encourage alternative behaviors for jealous clients—especially those that are anxiety-reducing in themselves (e.g., progressive relaxation or vigorous exercise). But particularly show them that they can stand experiencing some anxiety about their partner's whereabouts and that they do not *need* to seek immediate relief by spying on their partners or confronting them. Thus, through behavioral interventions, you help clients change their cognitions ("I *must* know what my partner is doing!") and to dispute their low frustration tolerance that has led to compulsive jealous actions.

Sometimes you discover jealous reactions that do not involve romantic rivals, but some activity or involvement that detracts from one partner's dependence on the other. Here again the restricted mate may come to feel stifled, and the couple may come to therapy. As with romantic jealousy, you look for thinking leading to insecurity, such as a jealous partner believing, "I must be validated by my mate's total attention!" Or "I cannot be safe or happy by myself, but absolutely *need* my mate's undivided devotion!"

You can also work with the *partners* of highly jealous people. They often disturb themselves about their partner's overpossessiveness, yet not take any effective action. You can show them that they *define* their spouse's obnoxious, jealous behavior as "intolerable" and can see it, instead, as merely unfortunate. They can then see the most effective ways to either discourage the behavior or minimize its effects (including considering the alternative of leaving the relationship). Most clients want some tools for discouraging jealous excesses. Teach them nonreinforcement and giving the jealous spouse poor consequences for making married life difficult. Encourage spouses *not* to accommodate their own lives to the partner's unreasonable demands.

When spouses keep rewarding extreme possessiveness, look into their own irrational thinking. They may foolishly think that jealous displays reassure them that they are a desirable person. Or they may believe that they *can't stand* the jealous partner's false accusations and may therefore overly restrict their own lives. If so, reveal and dispute their irrationalities.

Sometimes the jealous partner wants the other to submit to endless questioning, but only is satisfied with incriminating answers. In such cases, suggest to the accused mate that he or she not cooperate in playing that game, but instead urge the jealous partner to have therapy sessions.

Often a couple will come to counseling after the jealous interactions have taken a considerable toll on the relationship. Then you can ask the nonjealous spouse to give you some time to help change the partner's beliefs and actions. And it may still be impossible to accomplish this, so that the most that can be hoped is that the plague of extreme jealousy can be avoided in future relationships.

Here is an example of part of an RET session with a jealous and angry couple:

Wife: [My husband] is always out. He's out running around. Probably with other women. There is no need for him to be out so much. He should want to be with me. I'm his wife.

Husband: What are you talking about? I'm not out that much.

Wife: But you don't deny being out with other women.

Husband: You're getting hysterical. I go out with the guys because I need to have outside interests. And your job is to keep the house together and be here when I get home.

Wife: Don't be so cavalier! Relationships are not supposed to be like this. We should always be together or at least as much as we can. If you are out with other women . . . Well, that would be it!

Therapist: You both seem to get pretty angry with each other.

Husband: Damn right. She has her duties and I have mine. She wants me to be someone I'm not. She should just accept her place and respect mine. It really gets to me after a while.

Therapist: [to wife] And you?

Wife: He gets me *so* angry I want to scream.

Therapist: You are both saying that your anger is caused by your partner. How is that?

[NOTE: At this point, both husband and wife go on to explain to the therapist several of the specific things that are done which make them angry. They are essentially asserting that their spouse's behaviors (As) cause them to feel the consequence of anger.

Therapist: You are both arguing that you each have no choice but to get angry. In other words, you believe your anger is uncontrollable and there is absolutely nothing you can do about it. You are saying that you can do nothing but get angry in response to your partner's behaviors.

Husband: No, but its' tough to ignore it.

Wife: Sometimes I am better than other times.

Therapist: While it is difficult to minimize your intense anger, sometimes you both do tend to manage it better than at other times?

Husband: Yes.

Wife: Yes.

Therapist: How do you account for the fact that sometimes you are really angry and other times you are only annoyed or even indifferent?

Wife: I try to make it less important and do things for myself. I try to just live my life.

Husband: I just forget about it. Or, I say it's not worth getting *so* damn angry. I'm going to give myself an ulcer or end up getting physical. No matter how pissed off I get, I don't want that.

Therapist: No, you don't. What you are both agreeing on is that your particular mood is really a function of the attributions you have about the relationship at any given time. When you "make it less important," your anger gets reduced. If you view "closeness" as an absolute need, you get more uptight. When you think *differently,* you in turn feel differently.

Husband: Yes. But am I just supposed to tolerate her demands on me?

Wife: And am I supposed to like the fact that we rarely have quality time together?

Therapist: The answer to both questions is "no." Although you want to both minimize your individual levels of anger so as to not only feel better but also to have a better shot at relating to each other, that is *not* to say that you want to work toward possibly accepting the things you don't like about each other.

Wife: I think we both get carried away at times. And, it does not get us anything except farther away from each other.

Husband: So how are we supposed to think? You can't just change the way you think about things with the snap of a finger.

Therapist: No, it's not *that* easy, but it can be done with some effort. First, we have to take a look at what is going on inside both of your heads that makes you both so upset.

Wife: What do you mean, "What is going on in my head?"

Therapist: If you were to get yourself really angry right now, how would you do it?

Wife: I'd think about my husband being out with other women. Like I said earlier, that would be it.

Therapist: That would be what?

Wife: The end of the line.

Therapist: What do you mean when you say "the end of the line?"

Wife: It would be terrible, and I wouldn't be able to tolerate it.

Therapist: [reflectively empathically] You are saying that it would be *awful* and *intolerable.*

Wife: Absolutely! It would be devastating, and I would not be able to tolerate it.

Husband: Are you threatening me with divorce? You have to learn that I have to have my space. And you have to understand. Women are supposed to stay home and care for their husbands and families. And I need that in a relationship.

[NOTE: Here it should be clear that the wife's requirements that a relationship be "closer" and her tendency to catastrophize her husband's "potential" affairs lead her not only to increasingly predict that he's out with other women, but to also cause her a disproportionate amount of anger and jealousy that is inappropriate. Similarly, the husband's cavalier and possessive attitude only feeds into her tendency toward distrust, anger, and jealousy.]

Therapist: [to husband] How do you get yourself emotionally charged?
Husband: By just thinking about our relationship.
Therapist: That's right. Your thinking is primarily responsible for making you so angry. But what do you specifically say to yourself to get yourself upset?
Husband: I just think about how she does not trust me or give me any space. I can't stand that about her. Husbands need space. And I need her there for me when I'm home. I don't need this crap that she gives me about "sharing" and "quality time."
Therapist: You both pretty much share a common idea. You both *believe* that a relationship *is supposed* to be a certain way. That is, you [wife] assert that there must be a great overlap in your lives, while you [husband] *require* there to be very little overlap. And you both believe that you *need* it to run your way.
Husband: That's right. I need a woman who will always be there and not always question me.
Wife: And I need a husband who will need me for me and not for what I can do for him. I need a *husband!* Not just a roommate. I need intimacy and greater closeness.
Therapist: Let's examine these so-called needs. [to wife] What do you mean when you say you *need* these things?
Wife: If the relationship is going to work, I need him to be more attentive.
Therapist: [reflectively] I understand that closeness can in fact help the relationship. It could really benefit you. But how does that translate into your absolutely *needing* it or him?
Wife: Because things would go more smoothly.
Therapist: I agree that they might. However, you keep telling me the reasons why greater closeness is *preferable* and *advantageous.* You have yet to tell me your reasons why you *need* them just because they might help the relationship.
Wife: Well, of course, I don't need things to be different. I don't need him either. In fact, I don't even care what he does any more. I'm fed up.

[NOTE: As is often the case, this client starts giving up her notion of *need* in favor of an often equally self-defeating apathetic attitude.]

Therapist: I don't think that you really "don't care."
Husband: Then I shouldn't care either.
Therapist: You are both misunderstanding the point. You can give up your "need" for something without going to the extreme of trying to believe you "don't care." Saying you "don't care" is just not true. Saying you "need" the relationship to have certain features is similarly not true. I want you to both see that you can still really care about something without thinking you *need,* or *absolutely must have* it.
Husband: I understand. But it is important *to me* to have a wife who takes care of me and the things around the house.
Therapist: Fine. But can you give up your dire *need* for something that you really *want?*
Husband: [laughing] Of course.

Wife: I see the point. But I have one problem with that.
Therapist: What's that?
Wife: I accept that I don't *need* the relationship to be a certain way just because I *want* it. But if I don't have a caring and sharing and loving mate, I will be incomplete.
Therapist: Incomplete? Meaning what?
Wife: It would prove that I am not an adequate person. I wouldn't be complete.
Therapist: Because your *marriage* wouldn't be complete or because your *life* may lack some preferred feature? How does that mean that *you* are not adequate? Although your life may have less than you prefer, how does that equate to *you* being *less* than okay?
Wife: [stammers] Uh . . .
Therapist: You don't have an answer?
Wife: No.
Therapist: What does that tell us?
Wife: There is no answer?
Therapist: Take away the question mark.
Wife: There is no answer!
Therapist: Which means . . .
Wife: [weakly] I am *not* incomplete just because my marriage might be?
Therapist: Is that a statement or a question?
Wife: A statement!
Therapist: Then, explain it to me more fully.
Wife: Well, I don't need anyone to fulfill my life. I would like to have a different kind of relationship, but I'm not going to die without it. And my worth is not, and I repeat, *is not* contingent upon the quality of my relationships.
Therapist: How do you feel now that you have given up your *neediness* and self-berating?
Wife: Not terrific. But I am less angry and in better control.
Therapist: Good. Now [to husband], let's go back to your need for space and your need to have your wife act in a certain way.
Husband: I said before. I don't *need* it, but I still really want it. [angrily] Who the hell does she think she is? A wife is *supposed* to follow her husband's direction!
Therapist: On one hand, you are saying that you don't *need* those things, and on the other hand, you say she's *supposed* to provide them.
Husband: Damn right. She's *my* wife.
Therapist: I don't understand why she *must*.
Husband: Because, like I said, wives are simply supposed to. That's how it is.
Therapist: You say that so absolutely, as if it were a Law of the Universe.
Husband: I don't care about the damn universe. I care about what my wife does and doesn't do.
Therapist: So, it's *your* law.
Husband: Yeah. Well . . . it's not a *law*.
Therapist: When you get yourself angry, aren't you thinking of it as a law that she must obey?
Husband: I guess. But I don't mean it that way.
Therapist: How do you mean it?

Husband: I would really hope that she would give me some space and do more "feminine" things.

Therapist: Now you sound less angry. Why do you think that is?

Husband: Honestly? Because I guess I am a little less demanding.

Therapist: That's right. Let's approach this from another direction. Explain to me why she does not *have to* do what you want her to do.

Husband: Because she can make her own decisions. And I guess I really don't have to like them. I do want her to make changes in how she deals with me still. But she doesn't have to.

Therapist: You both gave up your beliefs that you *need* the relationship to run the way you individually *want* it to run. How might that affect your abilities to try to work things out?

Wife: More cooperatively probably. I get myself crazy.

Husband: And there's no reason to. I guess I play into it. It would be better if I just tell you more that "I love you" . . . and show it more. It's just that when I detect your anger and jealousy, I get distant.

Wife: Which makes me more jealous and suspicious.

Therapist: What makes you jealous and suspicious?

Wife: [laughs] *I* do.

Therapist: Right! By telling yourself what *should* or *must*?

Wife: Mmm. I don't really know.

Therapist: Yes, you do—if you merely look for it. But let me ask your husband. Do you see the *should* or *must* by which she makes herself intensely jealous?

Husband: I think so. "He, my husband, *must* only be interested in me—and in no other women.

Therapist: [to wife] Is he right?

Wife: Yes, I must *know* he will always be faithful to me.

Therapist: And if he isn't?

Wife: That makes me his infidelity, an unlovable, worthless person!

Therapist: Does it really make you *anything*, his infidelity?

Wife: No, I guess not. It merely makes *him* an unfaithful husband.

Therapist: Right—and it would not mean anything about you.

Husband: No, I can see what you mean. It would only mean something about me—about my tastes—and nothing necessarily about her.

Therapist: Right. Now, if I could only get both of you to strongly and persistently see that infidelity does not *cause* jealousy and self-downing and that only your own irrational ideas *do* lead to jealous feelings, you both would feel sorry and displeased, but *not* intensely jealous and insecure about the other's act or imagined outside affairs.

Wife: That would be great!

Husband: It certainly would be!

[NOTE: The therapist then summarized what the husband and wife were doing to make themselves angry and jealous and showed them how to keep monitoring and disputing their *need* and *must* beliefs and how to take activity homework—such as allowing the other to do things they didn't like—in order to practice feeling unangry and unjealous when they didn't get exactly what they wanted.]

Chapter 9
Effecting Marital Therapy Through Individual Therapy

Although most marital and family therapists today seem to espouse conjoint therapy with the main partners being seen together, and usually in the therapist's office at the same time, it is probable that the great majority of married people who are helped by therapy are largely seen in individual sessions, with their mates only occasionally seen conjointly. This is because most people who come for psychotherapy are driven to do so because of their own severe feelings of anxiety, depression, rage, and self-pity and because of their own behavioral problems (e.g., procrastination, overeating, drinking and drugging, phobias, obsessions, and compulsions). But people with these neurotic, borderline, and psychotic difficulties almost always have relationship troubles, and commonly handle their marital and family issues much better as a result of therapy, even when their mates are rarely or not seen by their therapist.

One of the pioneers in pointing out the limitations of conjoint marriage and family therapy is Robert A. Harper (1981), who also is the first therapist to join me (A.E.) in doing RET back in the 1950s and who has authored a number of seminal articles and books on RET (Harper, 1960; Ellis & Harper, 1961, 1975). He gives several important reasons why conjoint marriage and family therapy is often disadvantageous and why relationship problems had better often be handled by one therapist seeing both partners individually or, even better, by two separate therapists seeing both in individual sessions.

1. Conjoint therapy "tends to denigrate the importance of the individual" and to focus on an abstraction, "a marriage or a family or, in multiple family therapy, even a community of families" (Harper, 1981, p. 3).

98

2. "A focus on anything other than personal freedom and individual self-expression and self-actualization leads him or her quite subtly into a mild kind of totalitarianism in his or her orientation. I find the tendency to stress the primacy of *relationships*, and to treat psychopathology as if it resides in *intentions* rather than in *individuals*, oppositional to the personal philosophy and therapeutic ideology expressed so well by Erich Fromm three decades ago" (Harper, 1981, p. 3).

3. Good therapy requires that the therapist is accorded the full confidence and trust of the client, and this is only likely to be achieved in a one-to-one relationship.

4. When therapists see both partners conjointly, they frequently consciously or unconsciously favor one over the other and are therefore often not dealing fairly (or openly) with the unfavored mate.

Harper's pioneering views against the general obsession that family therapists have with conjoint sessions have been supported by similar objections by other writers, including Scheflin & Ferber (1972), Bowen (1978), and Allen (1988.) Stressing the importance of the self theories of Kohut (1971, 1977), Bowen (1978), and others, Allen (like Harper) stresses the conflict between the family system, with its biases for stability and homeostasis, with the healthy desires of family members to differentiate from the collective "in a process known as separation-individuation" (Allen, 1988, p. 354). To this end, he recommends that couples and family therapy be done largely in individual sessions with one or both partners.

When you use RET to see marital and family members individually, you can employ some of the following procedures.

Procedures for Treating Marital and Family Members Individually

Primary Client

Your primary client is usually one partner or member of the family. Your main goal is to help him or her overcome serious emotional and behavioral problems and to be a happier person, both within and outside of the marriage. Your main focus (unless the client chooses otherwise) is on helping the individual and not on perpetuating or abetting the marriage or the system. But since the individual inevitably lives within the system and is importantly affected by it, you also try to improve and modify the family system itself.

Marital Disturbance and Dissatisfaction

As noted throughout this book, you tackle both the client's emotional-behavioral disturbance *and* dissatisfaction. Because the former is often a prime causative factor of the latter, you especially try to help your individual clients acknowledge how disturbed they are and how they are largely creating their disturbances by holding irrational Beliefs (iBs) and persisting in inappropriate Consequences (iCs). You show them how to use several RET cognitive, emotive, and behavioral techniques to change these iBs and iCs (as indicated in Chapter 6).

At the same time, you investigate their marital (and other) dissatisfactions, and the practical problems that contribute to them, and you help the clients with problem solving, advice, planning, education, and skill training, to minimize their dissatisfactions and increase their family (and other) enjoyments.

Relationship with the Client

While following professional and ethical rules, you show real interest in helping your clients and serve as their friend, advisor, teacher, and encourager. You empathically try to see things from *their* frame of reference and usually go along with their goals and values, but by no means with their self-defeating *musts* and *commands* about achieving these values. You unconditionally accept your *clients* (as *persons*) while often rejecting and correcting their dysfunctional *behaviors*.

Clients' Influences on Others

Show your clients that they often importantly *influence* but not necessarily *disturb* other family members. Thus, a husband *frustrates* his wife by refusing to communicate with her, but he does not really *make her* enraged, since she has a choice of how to feel *about* his frustrating her. And the wife who criticizes her husband severely for not communicating with her *bothers* him with her nagging, but she does not really *make him* feel guilty and depressed. So you can often therapeutically show these mates how they *influence* and *affect* but not necessarily *disturb* each other.

Explain Partners' Disturbances

Using RET principles, show your individual clients exactly how their mates often disturb themselves by telling themselves irrational Beliefs and foolishly indulging in self-defeating habits. Show these clients how their mates are biologically and environmentally predisposed to be disturbed, how they unwittingly perpetuate and exacerbate their disturbances, and how they can often be helped by your clients to become more rational and self-helping. Encourage your clients constructively to teach RET methods to their spouses and children (Ellis, 1988b).

Explain Partners' Intentions

Your clients will often accuse their family members of deliberately, willfully harming them. If so, point out to them the likelihood that these "villains" are really emotionally disturbed and that their "deliberate" and "vicious" acts largely result from disturbances over which, at this time, they have relatively little control.

Uprooting Clients' Defensiveness

Your clients will frequently be defensive and will fail to acknowledge their own contributions to marital difficulties because they would damn themselves if they did acknowledge them. You can usually figure out, especially by talking to their spouses a few times, what some of the unacknowledged problems of your individual clients are and how these affect their marriages. Often, you can tactfully and undamningly bring these to your clients' attention, and they will then acknowledge and deal with them.

When they still resist, you can keep teaching them, generally and specifically, the RET philosophy that although many acts are foolish, unfortunate, or immoral, they are never stupid, bad, or rotten *people*. By helping them in this manner to feel unashamed and self-accepting, you will often be able to enable them to be less defensive and more open about their marital (and other) behavior and therefore more willing to change this behavior.

Dealing with Client's Anger and Rage

Many clients will admit their anger at their mates and their children when seen individually and not in joint sessions. Others will fight with their partners in joint sessions and become so angry that you, as therapist, will have great difficulty in getting them to look at what they are telling themselves to make themselves angry and to change these iBs. Seeing such clients individually, and sometimes seeing them for a number of sessions, often works much better than conjoint therapy. In one of my (A.E.'s) recent cases, I saw a fifty-year-old male mainly because of his twenty-five-year history of fighting with his wife (which four years of previous psychoanalytic therapy had not interrupted). After twelve sessions of RET, his wife noticed so much improvement in his bellicosity that she (a therapist herself) also came to see me for individual sessions. Soon after fights were almost nonexistent—largely because I kept strongly showing both of them, individually, how they were foolishly enraging themselves and blaming the other for being hostile. I find that partners who are very angry at their mates are often best treated in individual RET sessions. It is much better for them to fight with me about their hostility-creating nonsense than to keep fighting with each other.

Dealing with Clients' Enabling and Misguided Altruism

As Alcoholics Anonymous has pointed out for many years, and as some family therapists have noted, many partners unassertively overlook their mate's failings and altruistically enable them to continue their addictive, compulsive, and other self-sabotaging behavior. Or, conversely, they incessantly nag about this behavior and thereby encourage their partners to continue it rebelliously (Allen, 1988). Confronting such mates in conjoint sessions will frequently do more harm than good, but if you nondamningly get after them in individual therapy that is also maritally oriented, you may better be able to help them acknowledge their antimarital addictions and to change.

Abetting Individualism and Social Interest

Alfred Adler (1964a, 1964b) was a pioneering therapist who mainly worked with individual clients but was also a strong proponent of social interest. You, as an RET practitioner, can also favor marriage, family, and social interest while also encouraging individual health and well-being (Ellis, 1957, 1973a, 1988a; Ellis & Becker, 1982; Ellis & Dryden, 1987; Ellis & Harper, 1961). But since individualism, as noted at the beginning of this chapter, is sometimes neglected during conjoint family sessions, you can pay more attention to fostering it, while at the same time encouraging social interest, during individual sessions with family members. During such sessions, you can clearly push enlightened self-interest, but you can also show your clients that (1) they *are* an integral part of their family system; (2) if they sabotage this system, they also simultaneously defeat themselves; (3) when they help and satisfy other family members, they directly and indirectly abet their own enjoyments; (4) they teach RET more effectively to themselves when they use it and teach it to other individuals in the family system.

Allen(1988, p. 266) has nicely summarized the goal of family therapy and helping clients "to give up unnecessary and destructive aspects of their persons and to express their true selves, while remaining in close, helpful contact with their families." You can help clients do this in conjoint sessions, but, paradoxically, you can sometimes help them do it better in individual therapy sessions.

Experimenting with Love and Kindness

When partners insist that their mates are treating them unfairly and unlovingly, you can sometimes assume that they are correct about their perceptions (even when you suspect that they are exaggerating) and say something like this:

"Let's assume that you are right and that your spouse is overly critical and unloving. Being nasty in return will get the two of you nowhere—as I think you are already seeing—and hardly gets you the affection you crave. Now, instead, why don't you try being warm for the next few weeks? No matter how badly your partner treats you, lean over backwards to be very nice and loving in return. Do your best to be very warm and accepting. Try this, really try for the next few weeks. No matter how 'undeserving' you think your partner is, try being warm and loving—try for *your* sake. For by doing so you will soon see that your mate improves and begins to treat you much better—or you will see no improvement and continued cold and hostile behavior. If you get love and warmth, that will be fine. If you see no improvement, that will be fine, too. For you then will see that nothing that you do really works and that your mate really doesn't care or has very serious problems showing love and fairness. You can then decide what you can do about that—including probably separating. So you have everything to gain and nothing to lose by this experiment. Try it for a few weeks and see!" (Ellis, 1988b).

By inducing one of the partners (or sometimes both of them, individually) to try this experiment in being warm and kind to a supposedly unloving mate, you and your clients can discover some important information about themselves and their mates—especially about their own and their spouse's low frustration tolerance!

Communication and Skill Training

As noted in Chapter 6, skill training in general and communication training in particular is an important part of RET. Family members, when they start to surrender their irrational Beliefs and the disturbed Consequences that flow from them, still may not know how to assert themselves and to communicate with each other adequately. Such skills can be taught in conjoint sessions but, especially where one spouse is notably deficient, can often be more effectively taught and practiced in individual sessions with family members.

Disputation Problems

Conjoint therapy sessions, like RET group therapy sessions, have the advantage of family members hearing you actively dispute one person's irrational Beliefs and thereby realizing that they themselves hold these same ideas and that, as you are showing, they are invalid and destructive. But when one member of the family sticks solidly to his or her iBs despite your Disputing, the others may denigrate the rigid client and use his or her irrationality to "prove" that they are right and the irrational one is wrong about many other family affairs. Rigid partners, therefore, are often best dealt with in individual sessions, in the course of which you can vigorously Dispute their iBs without favoring the other partner. The presence of another family member during an intensive session with a difficult mate or child may also sidetrack the conversation and dilute the good work that you might otherwise be able to do with this difficult person.

Handling Difficult Partners

In many instances, you will find that one mate is relatively sane and sensible while the other is not. Thus, one spouse may be psychotic, addicted to drugs or alcohol, continually argumentative, cruel to the couple's children, a compulsive liar, or an inveterate gambler. Such a partner could well use therapy but refuses to come for it, to have his or her own therapist, or resents you dealing with his or her own problems in conjoint sessions. The best you may be able to do in these instances is to work with the other partner to help him or her become undisturbed *about* the other's behavior and to learn how to cope with it more effectively. In such cases, you may see both partners individually. But at times, especially if you have personal distastes for the actions of the difficult partner, it may be best to work only with that individual and show him or her how to survive better in a troublesome relationship that he or she doesn't want to end (Ellis, 1988b).

Divorce Situations

Couples frequently have emotional and practical problems about separation and divorce, and you can sometimes help them significantly in this respect and show them how to separate amicably. But because of legal battles and other reasons, conjoint sessions may not work out, and you and one of the partners may be better off with individual sessions in which you help this partner to cope with the separation problems. Showing one partner how to refuse to upset himself or herself about divorce proceedings may considerably aid both spouses to settle their differences more amicably.

Summary

For a number of reasons, as just shown, you or your clients may decide that it is more feasible to see one of them for regular individual rather than joint sessions about their marital or family dissatisfactions and disturbances. If so, remember that there is nothing sacred about having joint sessions, although they are often desirable. Be flexible in this regard! Thus, you can usually see couples together—and occasionally see each of them separately. Or you can usually see only one family member—and can occasionally see the others conjointly. Or you can see the parents together and the children by themselves. Or, in exceptional cases (e.g., where one mate is paranoid), you can insist on only seeing one of the partners. There are many possible variations, and you may sometimes use one and sometimes another.

At times, you may be forced to use either conjoint or individual sessions—as when one mate refuses to come for therapy or when one refuses to come unless the other is also present. If so, do the best you can and remember that most RET techniques, especially the Disputing of irrational Beliefs, can best be done with either or both mates present but that they also can be adapted to less optimal conditions. Because you are attempting, by using RET, to help your marital and family clients to be less rigid and more flexible, try to model flexibility yourself in your contacts with them.

Chapter 10

A Rational-Constructivist Approach to Couples and Family Therapy

Several leading cognitive therapists have recently held that there are two distinct kinds of cognitive-behavioral therapy: (1) the "rationalist" approach, which adopts a surface-associationist model, typified by the theories and practices of Beck (1976), Ellis (1962), Goldfried and Davison (1976), and Meichenbaum (1977); and (2) the deep-structure "constructivist" approach, which is typified by the writings of Guidano (1988), Guidano & Liotti (1983), Mahoney (1988), and Reda and Mahoney (1984). Assuming that this distinction is to some degree valid, it clearly does not hold for rational-emotive therapy, which the "constructivists" wrongly put in the "rationalist" camp (Ellis, 1989).

If "constructivist" cognitive therapies truly can be differentiated from "rationalist" therapies, RET is perhaps the most constructivist and most deep structurist of the present-day popular therapies. In regard to couples and family therapy, as has been shown in the previous chapters of this book, RET is unusually rational in that it shows clients what are their irrational, unrealistic, illogical, and antiscientific cognitions and how to use thinking, feeling, experiential, and behavioral methods to change them. But rational-emotive couples therapy is also unusually constructivist and some of its constructivist aspects will now be briefly summarized.

CONSTRUCTIVIST ASPECTS OF RATIONAL-EMOTIVE COUPLES THERAPY

Deep Cognitive Structures

In rational-emotive couples therapy, therapists do not merely try to identify clients' unrealistic views of and illogical conceptions about "reality," but also attempt to reveal their underlying, often unconscious, basic disturbance-creating philosophies—especially their dogmatic, rigid, grandiose musts, shoulds, oughts, demands, and commands. They are shown how to arrive at, as Guidano puts it, "alternate models of the self and the world such that the deep structures can adopt a more flexible and adaptive articulation" (1988, p. 306). Instead of mainly trying to change the family system, and thereby induce change in its members, RET tries to help all family members make a profound philosophic change—as well as also change the system in which they participate (Ellis, 1985a, 1988a; Ellis & Dryden, 1987).

Tacit and Explicit Levels of Knowing

RET holds that while marital and family members largely imbibe their conscious or explicit goals, standards, and values from significant others in their early lives, they rarely disturb themselves merely by these explicit rules and preferences. Rather, they innately and implicitly *create* and *construct* (rather than just *learn*) underlying, deeply structured dogmas that they put on themselves, on others, and on the world *about* their imbibed rules. RET couples therapy is one of the few systems of treatment that specifically seeks out, reveals, and shows clients how to change their deeply structured implicit dogmas—and how, ideally, to reduce their tendencies toward dogma-making and to enhance their innate tendencies to think more flexibly and scientifically (Ellis, 1962, 1987a, 1987b, 1988a; Ellis & Dryden, 1987).

Attachment Process and Self-Identity

Guidano and Liotti (1983; Guidano, 1988), following Bowlby (1969, 1973) stress the importance of the attachment process in children and its influence on the achievement of self-identity. RET largely agrees with this theory, but particularly shows that children have a strong biological tendency to *create* attachments to their parents and other family members and also to take their strong preferences for affection and love (which are both inborn and acquired) and transmute them into dire necessities. According to rational-emotive therapy, it is not the *lack* or *loss* of parental love itself that makes children lose identity and become depressed, but it is largely children's view of that loss or lack, which they partly construct. RET marriage and family therapy emphasizes showing family members how to keep their preferences but surrender their dire needs for approval and affection, to thereby differentiate themselves from their families—as Allen (1988) and Bowen (1978) also encourage—and to achieve a greater degree of unconditional, *self*-identity or *self*-acceptance (Ellis, 1972c, 1973a, 1988a; Ellis & Dryden, 1987).

Personal Identity and Self-Evaluation

Guidano states that personality identity "is fundamentally an inferred knowledge of oneself, biased by one's own tacit self-knowledge" (1988, p. 317). RET couples therapy more specifically assumes that people are born with tendencies to tacitly (and explicitly) rate, first, their performances and traits and, second, their personal identities or "selves." *Self*-rating is an over generalization, is often pernicious, and easily leads to self–damnation—which is one of the prime causes of marital and family dissatisfaction and disturbance. RET holds, more than virtually all the other forms of therapy, and more than Guidano, Mahoney, Reda, Liotti, and other cognitive constructivists, that self-evaluations are sometimes influenced by and accepted from one's parents and siblings, but that they are largely tacitly invented and constructed because of people's innate predisposition to take other's ratings of their performances and change them into ratings of their selves (Ellis, 1972c, 1973a, 1976b, 1988a).

Models of Reality

Mahoney (1988) and other constructivists hold that the human mind is an active system that imposes order on the environment and that "it is not the 'real' world but how it is construed that plays the crucial role and the ongoing tacit ordering of life events into personal meanings is primary" (Guidano, 1988, p. 32). RET has posited a similar view of "reality" since its beginnings in 1955 (Ellis, 1957, 1962). It shows people in couples therapy that Activating Events (As) *contribute* to disturbed Consequences (Cs) but that their mate's Belief Systems (Bs) largely *create* or *cause* these Consequences (Ellis, 1962, 1973a, 1978c, 1985a, 1988a). RET also shows clients in family therapy that the relationships between A, B, and C are not linear but circular and that just as cognitions influence feelings and behaviors, so do the latter influence thoughts and affect each other (Ellis, 1958a, 1962, 1985a, 1985b, 1988a; Ellis & Dryden, 1987). So RET, although in some ways significantly different from what is usually called systems family therapy, is in its own right a pioneering form of systems therapy.

Life-span Development

Following Hayek (1978), Guidano (1988) sees conscious rationality stemming from people's life experiences and how they interpret these interests and deal with them, rather than stemming from human design. RET takes an even more constructivist position and holds that family members are born with strong predispositions toward (conscious and unconscious) creativity and design. Humans can *deliberately* design their own changes and seem to have more "free will" and conscious decision making than Hayek and Guidano are willing to grant them. RET encourages and teaches couples how to use their underlying creativity to achieve more satisfying, less stereotyped relationships.

Approaches to Truth and Reality

Guidano places RET in an empirical-associationist camp and states that it considers truth "singular, static, and external to all humans" (1988, p. 326). And he holds that in constructivist therapy, clients' basic assumptions underlying their way of experiencing reality "are viewed as being in need of modification not because they are irrational but because they represent an outmoded solution."

Guidano misrepresents RET, for as Ellis has clearly stated, "RET posits no absolutist or invariant criteria of rationality" and "RET therapists do *not* select clients' values, goals, and purposes or show them what their basic aims and purposes *should* be" (Ellis & Whiteley, 1979, p. 40). RET defines people's experience of "reality" as "irrational" only when they create or construct thoughts, feelings, and behaviors that often defeat or sabotage their *own, personal* goals, values, and interests. In RET, "irrational" mainly means self-defeating and "rational" means providing better solutions to marital problems than couples have yet devised. RET also sees family members as largely constructing or inventing the "reality" of their childhood and current "experiences" and then bigotedly *accepting* these "experiences" as "truths." Where Guidano seems to think that because these experiences existed and were deeply felt they *are* "true," RET takes a more relativist and constructionist attitude about their "reality" and their "truth."

The Role of Developmental Analysis

Mahoney (1988) and Guidano (1988, p. 328) take a heavily psychoanalytic position and hold that "any distortion of the patterns of family attachment will be reflected in the child's developing self-identity." RET family therapy assumes, instead, that the child's developing self-identity is significantly *correlated with* but hardly completely *dependent on* patterns of family attachment. RET holds that the child is heavily *influenced* but not *disorganized* by family attachments and that its identity disorders largely stem from its *reactions*, on a heavily individualized basis, to these patterns. Where Guidano's and Mahoney's position is more of a stimulus-response position of psychoanalysts and orthodox behaviorists, the RET position is much more of a stimulus-organism-response theory and is more constructivist.

Clients Resistance to Change

Guidano (1988, p. 329) attributes most client resistance to therapists being too active-directive, to not forming a deep collaborative working alliance with their clients, and to their taking a too "reasonable" attitude that is threatening to clients' already constructed models of themselves and others. This is questionable in regard to couples therapy, as a large number of marital and family therapists have shown that behavioral, strategic planning, problem solving, skill training, and other active-directive methods have often worked very well (Allen, 1988; Burns, 1984; Ellis, 1977a, 1984a, 1985a; Grieger, 1988; Haley, 1976; Hauck, 1977; Huber & Baruth, 1989; Jacobson & Margolin, 1979; Kanfer & Schefft, 1988; A. A. Lazarus, 1985; Sager, 1976; Stuart, 1980). RET assumes that people in a marital and family system largely train themselves to become disturbed and to disrupt the system; that they reinforce themselves to feel relatively comfortable with and to hold on to their dissatisfactions and disturbances; and that they consciously and unconsciously *hang on* to the self-defeating thoughts, feelings, and behaviors that they create. Therefore, effective couples therapists had better actively show their clients what they are now doing and actively directively teach them how to overcome their resistance to change (Ellis, 1985a; Kanfer & Schefft, 1988). RET, as shown in Chapter 6, is also more emotive, experiential, evocative, and dramatic than are most cognitive-behavioral couples therapies.

Superficial and Deep Changes

Guidano prides himself on helping clients make deep rather than superficial changes and notes that "a superficial change coincides with the reorganization of the client's attitude toward reality without revising his or her personality" (1988, p. 330). Guidano seems to be referring here to the "superficial" therapy of Beck (1976), Meichenbaum (1977), and other cognitive therapists who largely help clients to change their inferences and misperceptions about reality (e.g., "Because my mate criticizes my sex performance, she hates me totally and that means that I'll *never* be good at sex or at relating"). RET agrees with Guidano and Mahoney that this is somewhat superficial cognitive therapy and, instead, seeks out the profound, commanding, musturbatory philosophy that usually creates these reality distortions (e.g., "Because I *must* always do well sexually and win my mate's total approval, and because she is now criticizing me sexually, I am sure that she hates me *totally* and that means I'll *never* be good at sex or at relating!"). RET, as shown in this book, tries to have all the family members achieve a profound philosophic and personality change rather than merely a superficial change in their perceptions of reality; and it is probably more constructivist in this respect than the therapies of Guidano, Mahoney, and other cognitive constructivists.

Strategy for Therapeutic Change

Following the therapy rules outlined by Bowlby in a July 1982 personal communication to him, Guidano insists that an effective cognitive therapist must show clients how they got the cognitive models they subscribe to from their parents, how to review them in the light of their parental history, and how to recognize the sanctions their parents have used to insist that they adopt these parental models. This psychoanalytically oriented method assumes that people almost entirely become disturbed because of the influence of their parents and of their own early first-hand experiences with these influences. The RET approach, however, assumes that children bring their individual *selves* to their parental influences and that they therefore *interpret* these influences quite uniquely and differently and thereby *construct* much of their own *reactions* to parental teachings. RET individual and family therapy therefore largely reveals to clients not what their parents and families did to supposedly *mold* them but how they *constructed* their disturbed attitudes *about* their childhood environment. More importantly, RET shows clients how they are still, today, *inventing* self-defeating beliefs and behaviors.

RET strategy for therapeutic change is therefore distinctly more constructiveist than the Bowlby–Guidano strategy.

Guidano insists that as it is the clients' tacit self-knowledge that makes them capable of revising their cognitive models in already available ways, and only has to be brought to their attention, "it is useless and even dangerous to put new knowledge into the client's head in every possible way, since the information useful for the client comes from his or her deep structure and cannot be replaced by the therapist's conceptions about life" (1988, p. 332).

This follows the psychoanalytic notion that people unconsciously become disturbed and only have to *see* or *gain insight* into their unconscious thoughts to automatically change them. But the last hundred years of individual and family therapy has fairly conclusively shown that insight is far from enough and that clients had better not only become aware of their thinking, as Guidano advocates, but also do a great deal of work to consciously change their cognitive models. Effective cognitive-behavioral therapists — as shown in RET couples therapy — do not replace their clients' concepts with their own concepts about life but do give these clients considerable new knowledge — and even some advice at times — about more scientific and less self-defeating ways of thinking, feeling, and behaving. RET practitioners present this new knowledge tentatively and experimentally, never as dogma, and give clients a *choice* of using it, modifying it, or ignoring it (Ellis & Dryden, 1987).

Guidano insists that therapists have to respect their clients' tacit level of thinking. "For example, it is useless and dangerous to try to convince individuals with depressive organizations that their inner view of themselves is absurd or to criticize their basic feelings about loneliness, ephemerality, and the futility of life. In some ways, these are the only possibilities they have of establishing the relationship with reality" (1988, p. 333).

This is quite an anticonstructivist notion, as it says that once people develop a negative view of themselves and of life, their "essential directionality" *has to* be respected and followed by therapists. RET holds, instead, that clients choose futile attitudes toward themselves and life, that they can *choose* to change, and that they can *choose* to follow their therapist's active-directive teachings. A great many studies have shown that RET and other cognitive-behavioral active interventions result in clients changing their inner view of themselves and becoming significantly less depressed (Beck, Rush, Shaw, & Emery, 1979; DiGiuseppe, Miller, & Trexler, 1979; Ellis & Whiteley, 1979a; Engels & Diekstra, 1988; Haaga & Davison, 1989; McGovern & Silverman, 1984).

Integration of Deep Cognition, Emotion, and Behavior

Mahoney states that cognitive constructivists hold that "acting, feeling, and knowing are inseparable expressions of adaptation and development" (1988, p. 370). He is correct about this, but significantly forgets that the same point has been clearly made in RET since 1956, before he and Guidano entered the field of psychotherapy (Ellis, 1958a, 1962). Ellis stated: "The theoretical foundations of RET are based on the assumption that human thinking and emotion are *not* two disparate or different processes, but that they significantly overlap and are in some respects, for all practical purposes, essentially the same thing. Like the other two basic life processes, sensing and moving, they are integrally interrelated and never can be seen wholly apart from each other" (1962, p. 38).

RET family therapy, as shown throughout this book, not only is highly cognitive but also unusually emotive and behavioral (see Chapter 6). Unlike most other cognitive-behavioral therapies, it emphasizes the close relationship between "hot" cognitions and emotions and therefore consistently uses a variety of dramatic, evocative, forceful verbal and action-oriented techniques.

Mahoney holds that "rationalist" therapies denigrate emotions and that these therapies claim that "all intensive emotions (regardless of valence) have a disorganizing effect on behavior" (1988, p. 374). It is not clear what "rationalist" therapies he is referring to in this criticism, but RET has never been opposed to intense emotions (e.g., strong feelings of sadness, disappointment, and grief) but only to disruptive, self-defeating emotions (e.g., panic, depression, and self-hatred). Unlike most other therapies, RET clearly distinguishes between *appropriate* and *in*appropriate feelings (Ellis, 1957, 1962, 1971, 1973a, 1977a, 1987a, 1988a; Ellis & Becker, 1982; Ellis & Dryden, 1987; Ellis & Harper, 1975). RET couples therapy often helps people to feel *more* strongly than they do when they first come to counseling—but not to feel just for the sake of feeling. And it emphasizes the enhancement of self-actualizing, happy feelings and not merely the elimination of destructive ones.

Therapeutic Relationship

Guidano (1988) and Mahoney (1988) (along with Freud [1965] and Rogers [1961]) stress the importance of the therapeutic relationship for personality change, and they wrongly assume that RET and other cognitive therapies ignore this aspect. On the contrary, as again shown in this book, RET particularly stresses that therapists had better always give individual and family clients unconditional acceptance or what Rogers calls unconditional positive regard; and that they not merely *tell* but *show* their clients that they are accepted by their therapists *whether or not* they perform adequately and *whether or not* they are nice and lovable. But in addition to *showing* and *modeling* unconditional acceptance, RET couples practitioners *teach* clients how to philosophically accept themselves, not because of but also independently of their therapist's acceptance (Ellis, 1973a, 1977a, 1988a; Ellis & Harper, 1975). This double-barreled RET approach uniquely emphasizes people's ability to choose and *construct* their own self-acceptance, and is therefore more constructionist than the psychoanalytically oriented approaches of Mahoney and Guidano.

Mahoney claims that classical "rationalists" see relapse and recidivism in therapy resulting from insufficient use of knowledge and information imparted during therapy while cognitive constructivists see setbacks and regression as "naturally and virtually inevitable aspects of psychological development" (1988, p. 378). Mahoney seems to forget that this position was clearly formulated in RET back in the 1960s (Ellis, 1962) and has been part and parcel of RET practice since that time (Ellis, 1973a, 1987c, 1988a; Ellis & Dryden, 1987). Unlike strategic and systems family therapy, RET assumes that family members not only largely *disturb themselves* about what happens to them in the family system but that they also consistently redisturb themselves even when a beneficial change in the system is arranged. As Ellis (1965b) has observed, people are born with a talent for defeating their own and their family's interest, *easily* do so, and *naturally* fall back to doing so again during the entire period of their lives.

If they profoundly change their basic, deep-seated, disturbance-creating philosophies, RET holds, and if they keep working to keep them flexible, they can often achieve the "elegant" solution of rarely (not *never*) upsetting themselves in the present and future and of quickly unupsetting themselves when they do fall back. So they have the ability, if they work hard at effective therapy, of making themselves *less* but not *non*upsettable (Ellis, 1987c). In this way, RET seems to be more constructivist than the cognitive therapies of Mahoney, Guidano, Reda, Liotti, and other cognitive constructivists.

CONCLUSION

Mahoney, Guidano, and other modern constructivists and process-oriented therapists are partly on the right track and are making some interesting additions to traditional cognitive therapy. But they sometimes also revert to inefficient and sidetracking psychoanalytically oriented methods of therapy. RET, in both its individual and family therapy approaches, attempts to use the most effective and hard-headed of the so-called rationalist methods—including active directive changing of unrealistic and irrational Beliefs, skill training, problem solving, bibliotherapy, in vivo desensitization, and reinforcement procedures—and it also employs many of the methods of the cognitive constructivists—including the disclosing of tacit philosophies, the achievement of a profound philosophical change in clients' attitudes toward themselves, toward others, and toward life situations, the use of the therapist's relationship with clients to show them how to unconditionally accept themselves, and the employment of many dramatic, emotive, and experiential exercises to change clients' feelings as well as their thoughts and behaviors. RET couples therapy is particularly interested in effecting both individual and familial change as quickly and as efficiently as feasible. It is therefore rational (efficaciously hedonic) *and* emotive (energetically experiential). Or at least tries to be!

REFERENCES

Adler, A. (1964a). *Superiority and social interests*, ed. by H. L. Ansbacker & R. R. Ansbacher. Evanston, IL: Northwestern University Press.

Adler, A. (1964b). *Social interest: A challenge to mankind*. New York: Capricorn.

Allen, D. M. (1988). Unifying individual and family therapies. San Francisco: Jossey-Bass.

Barbach, L. (1975). *For yourself: The fulfillment of female sexuality*. Garden City, NY: Doubleday.

Bard, J. (1980). *Rational-emotive therapy in practice*. Champaign, IL: Research Press.

Bard, J. (1987). *I don't like asparagus*. Cleveland, OH: Psychology Department, Cleveland State University.

Bass, B. A., & Walen, S. R. (1986). Rational-emotive treatment for the sexual problems of couples. *Journal of Rational-Emotive Therapy, 4*(1), 82–94.

Beck, A. T. (1976). *Cognitive therapy and the emotional disorders*. New York: International Universities Press.

Beck, A. T. (1988). *Love is never enough*. New York: Harper & Row.

Beck, A. T., Rush, A. J., Shaw, B. F., & Emery, G. (1979). *Cognitive therapy of depression*. New York: Guilfold.

Bernard, M. E. (1986). *Staying alive in an irrational world: Albert Ellis and rational-emotive therapy*. South Melbourne, Australia: Carlson/Macmillan.

Bernard, M. E., & Joyce, M. R. (1984). *Rational-emotive therapy with children and adolescents*. New York: Wiley.

Berne, E. (1972). *What do you say after you say hello?* New York: Grove.

Bowen, M. (1978). *Family therapy in clinical practice*. New York: Aronson.

Bowlby, J. (1969). *Attachment and loss, I: Attachment*. New York: Basic.

Bowlby, J. (1973). *Attachment and loss, II: Separation*. New York: Basic.

Burns, D. D. (1980). *Feeling good: The new mood therapy*. New York: Morrow.

Burns, D. (1984): *Intimate connections*. New York: Morrow.

Danysh, J. (1974). *Stop without quitting*. San Francisco: International Society for General Semantics.

DiGiuseppe, R. A., Miller, N. J., & Trexyler, L. D. (1979). A review of rational-emotive therapy outcome studies. In A. Ellis & M. Whiteley (eds.), *Theoretical and empirical foundations of rational-emotive therapy* (pp. 218–235). Monterey, CA; Brooks/Cole.

Dryden, W. (1984). *Rational-emotive therapy: Fundamentals and innovations*. Beckenham, Kent: Croom-Helm.

Ellis, A. (1954). *The American sexual tragedy*. New York: Twayne and Grove Press. Rev. ed., New York: Lyle Stuart and Grove Press, 1962.

Ellis, A. (1957). *How to live with a "neurotic": At home and at work.* New York: Crown. Rev. ed., North Hollywood, CA: Wilshire Books, 1975.

Ellis, A. (1958a). Rational psychotherapy. *Journal of General Psychology, 59,* 35–49. Reprinted; New York: Institute for Rational-Emotive Therapy.

Ellis, A. (1958b). *Sex without guilt.* New York: Lyle Stuart. Rev. ed, New York: Lyle Stuart, 1965.

Ellis, A. (1960). *The art and science of love.* Secaucus, NJ: Lyle Stuart.

Ellis, A. (1962). *Reason and emotion in psychotherapy.* Secaucus, NJ: Citadel.

Ellis, A. (1963). *The treatment of borderline and psychotic individuals* Rev. ed, 1988. New York: Institute for Rational-Emotive therapy.

Ellis, A. (1965a). *Suppressed: Seven key essays publishers dared not print.* Chicago: New Classics House.

Ellis, A. (1965b). Workshop on rational-emotive therapy. New York City, September 8.

Ellis, A. (1969a). A weekend of rational encounter. *Rational Living, 4*(2), 1–8.

Ellis, A. (1969b). A cognitive approach to behavior therapy. *International Journal of Psychiatry, 8,* 896–900.

Ellis, A. (1971). *Growth through reason.* North Hollywood, CA: Wilshire Books.

Ellis, A. (1972a). *The civilized couple's guide to extramarital adventure.* New York: Wyden and Pinnacle Books.

Ellis, A. (1972b). *Conquering low frustration tolerance,* cassette recording. New York: Institute for Rational-Emotive Therapy.

Ellis, A. (1972c). *Psychotherapy and the value of a human being.* New York: Institute for Rational-Emotive Therapy.

Ellis, A. (1973a). *Humanistic psychotherapy: The rational-emotive approach.* New York: McGraw-Hill.

Ellis, A. (Speaker). (1973b). *How to stubbornly refuse to be ashamed of anything,* cassette recording. New York: Institute for Rational-Emotive Therapy.

Ellis, A. (Speaker). (1973c). *Twenty-one ways to stop worrying,* cassette recording. New York: Institute for Rational-Emotive Therapy.

Ellis, A. (Speaker). (1975a). *Demonstration with a family,* videotape. New York: Institute for Rational-Emotive Therapy.

Ellis, A. (Speaker). (1975b). *How to be happy though mated,* cassette recording. New York: Institute for Rational-Emotive Therapy.

Ellis, A. (1975c). (Speaker). *Solving emotional problems,* cassette recording. New York: Institute for Rational-Emotive Therapy.

Ellis, A. (Speaker). (1975d). *Interview with a man with fear of failure in love relations,* videotape. New York: Institute for Rational-Emotive Therapy.

Ellis, A. (1976a). *Sex and the liberated man.* Secaucus, NJ: Lyle Stuart.

Ellis, A. (1976b). RET abolishes most of the human ego. *Psychotherapy, 13,* 343–348. Reprinted, New York: Institute for Rational-Emotive Therapy.

Ellis, A. (Speaker). (1976c). *Conquering low frustration tolerance,* cassette recording. New York: Institute for Rational-Emotive Therapy.

Ellis, A. (1977a). *Anger—How to live with and without it.* Secaucus, NJ: Citadel Press.

Ellis, A. (Speaker). (1977b). *Dealing with sexuality and intimacy,* cassette recording. New York: BMA Audio Cassettes.

Ellis, A. (Speaker). (1977c). *Conquering the dire need for love,* cassette recording. New York: Institute for Rational-Emotive Therapy.

Ellis, A. (1977d). Fun as psychotherapy. *Rational Living, 12*(1), 2–6.

Ellis, A. (Speaker). (1977e). *A garland of rational humorous songs,* cassette recording, and songbook. New York: Institute for Rational-Emotive Therapy.

Ellis, A. (Speaker). (1978a). *I'd like stop but . . . Dealing with addictions,* cassette recording. New York: Institute for Rational-Emotive Therapy.

Ellis, A. (1978b). A rational approach to divorce problems. In S. M. Goetz (ed.), *Breaking asunder,* (pp. 27–33. Greenvale, NY: Therapist Center, Long Island University.

Ellis, A. (1978c). Family therapy: A phenomenological *and* active-directive approach. *Journal of Marriage and Family Counseling, 4*(2), 43–50. Reprinted, New York: Institute for Rational-Emotive Therapy.

Ellis, A. (1978d). Rational-emotive guidance. In L. E. Arnold (ed.)., *Helping parents help their children,* pp. 91–101. New York: Brunner/Mazel.

Ellis, A. (1979a). *The intelligent woman's guide to dating and mating.* Secaucus, NJ: Lyle Stuart.

Ellis, A. (1979b). Discomfort anxiety: A new cognitive behavioral construct. Part 1. *Rational Living, 14*(2), 3–8.

Ellis, A. (1980a). Discomfort anxiety: A new cognitive behavioral construct. Part 2. *Rational Living, 15*(1), 25–30.

Ellis, A. (1980b). Rational-emotive therapy and cognitive behavior therapy: Similarities and differences. *Cognitive Therapy and Research, 4,* 325–340.

Ellis, A. (1980c). The rational-emotive approach to children's and adolescents' sex problems. In J. M. Sampson (ed.), *Childhood and sexuality,* (pp. 513–524). Montreal, Canada: Edition Etudes Vivantes.

Ellis, A. (1980d). The treatment of erectile dysfunction. In S. R. Leiblum & A. L. Pervin (eds.), *Principles and practice of sex therapy,* (pp. 240–258). New York: Guildford.

Ellis, A. (Speaker). (1981). *Intelligent person's guide to dating and mating,* cassette recording. New York: Institute for Rational-Emotive Therapy.

Ellis, A. (1982). Rational-emotive family therapy. In A. M. Horne & M. M. Ohlsen (eds.), *Family counseling and therapy* pp. 302–328. Itasca, IL: Peacock.

Ellis, A. (1983). Rational-emotive therapy (RET) approaches to overcoming resistance. 1: Common forms of resistance. *British Journal of Cognitive Psychotherapy, 1*(1), 28–38.

Ellis, A. (1984a). Jealousy: Its etiology and treatment. In D. G. Goldberg (ed.), *Contemporary marriage,* pp. 420–438. Homewood, Il: Dorsey.

Ellis, A. (1984b). *Rational-emotive therapy intensive.* New York: Institute for Rational-Emotive Therapy, April 4.

Ellis, A. (1985a). *Overcoming resistance: Rational-emotive therapy with difficult clients.* New York: Springer.

Ellis, A. (1985b). Expanding the ABC's of rational-emotive therapy. In M. Mahoney & A. Freeman (eds.), *Cognition and psychotherapy* pp. 313–323. New York: Plenum.

Ellis, A. (1986a). Rational-emotive therapy applied to relationship therapy. *Journal of Rational-Emotive Therapy,* 4–21.

Ellis, A. (1986b). Anxiety about anxiety: The use of hypnosis with rational-emotive therapy. In E. T. Dowd & J. M. Healy (eds.), *Case studies in hypnotherapy,* pp. 3–11. New York: Guilford.

Ellis, A. (1987a). A sadly neglected cognitive element in depression. *Cognitive Therapy and Research, 11,* 121–146.

Ellis, A. (1987b). The use of rational humorous songs in psychotherapy. In W. F. Fry, Jr. & W. A. Salameh (eds.), *Handbook of humor and psychotherapy,* pp. 265–286. Sarasota, FL: Professional Resource Exchange.

Ellis, A. (1987c). The impossibility of achieving consistently good mental health. *American Psychologist, 42,* 364–375.

Ellis, A. (1987d). The evolution of rational-emotive therapy (RET) and cognitive behavior therapy (CBT). In J. K. Zeig (ed.), *The evolution of psychotherapy.* (pp. 107–133). New York: Brunner/Mazel.

Ellis, A. (1988a). *How to stubbornly refuse to make yourself miserable about anything—yes, anything!* Secaucus, NJ: Lyle Stuart.

Ellis, A. (1988b). How to live with a neurotic man. *Journal of Rational-Emotive and Cognitive-Behavior Therapy, 6,* 129–136.

Ellis, A. (1989). Is rational-emotive therapy (RET) "rationalist" or "constructivist"? Keynote address to the World Congress of Cognitive Therapy, Oxford, England, June 29. Also in A. Ellis & W. Dryden (1989), *The essential Albert Ellis.* New York: Springer.

Ellis, A., & Abrahams, E. (Speakers). (1978). *Brief psychotherapy and crisis intervention,* cassette recordings. New York: Institute for Rational-Emotive Therapy.

Ellis, A., & Becker, I. (1982). *A guide to personal happiness.* North Hollywood, CA: Wilshire Books.

Ellis, A., & Conway, R. O. (1967). *The art of erotic seduction.* New York: Lyle Stuart.

Ellis, A., & Bernard, M. E. (eds.). (1983): *Rational-emotive approaches to the problems of childhood,* New York: Plenum.

Ellis, A., & Bernard, M. E. (eds.). (1985). *Clinical applications of rational-emotive therapy.* New York: Plenum.

Ellis, A., & Dryden, W. (1987). *The practice of rational-emotive therapy.* New York: Springer.

Ellis, A., & Grieger, R. (eds.). (1977). *Handbook of rational-emotive therapy,* Vol. 1. New York: Springer.

Ellis, A., & Grieger, R. (eds.). (1986). *Handbook of rational-emotive therapy,* Vol. 2. New York: Springer.

Ellis, A., & Harper, R. A. (1961). *A guide to successful marriage.* North Hollywood, CA: Wilshire Books.

Ellis, A., & Harper, R. A. (1975). *A new guide to rational living.* North Hollywood, CA: Wilshire Books.

Ellis, A., McInerney, J. F., DiGiuseppe, R., & Yeager, R. J. (1988). *Rational-emotive therapy with alcoholics and substance abusers.* New York: Pergamon.

Ellis, A., & Whiteley, J. M. (1979). *Theoretical and empirical foundations of rational-emotive therapy.* Monterey, CA: Brooks/Cole.

Ellis, A., & Yeager, R. (1989). *Why some therapies don't work: The dangers of transpersonal psychology.* Buffalo, NY: Prometheus.

Engels, G., & Diekstra, R. F. W. (1986). Meta-analysis of rational-emotive therapy outcome studies. In P. Eelen & O. Fontaine (eds.), *Behavior therapy: Beyond the conditioning framework* (pp. 121–140). Hillsdale, NJ: Erlbaum.

Epsteiin, N. (1986). Cognitive marital therapy: Multilevel assessment and intervention. *Journal of Rational-Emotive Therapy, 4,* 68–81.

Freud, S. (1965). *Standard edition of the complete psychological works of Sigmund Freud.* London: Hogarth.

Fry, W. F., Jr., & Salameh, W. A. (eds.). (1987). *Handbook of humor and psychotherapy.* Sarasota, FL: Professional Resource Exchange.

Fullner, H. (1983). A structural approach to unresolved mourning in single parent family systems. *Journal of Marital and Family Therapy, 9*(3), 259–269.

Garfinkel, P. E., & Garner, D. M. (1982). *Anorexia nervosa: A multidimensional perspective.* New York: Bruner/Mazel.

Goldfried, M. R., & Davison, G. C. (1976). *Clinical behavior therapy.* New York: Holt, Rinehart & Winston.

Golden, W., Dowd, E. T., & Friedberg, F. (1987). *Hypnotherapy: A modern approach.* New York: Pergamon.

Greenwald, H. (1981). *Direct decision therapy.* San Diego, CA: Edits.

Grieger, R. (1986). The role and treatment of irresponsibility in dysfunctional relationships. *Journal of Rational-Emotive Therapy, 4*, 50–67.

Grieger, R. (ed.). (1988) *Rational-emotive couples therapy*. New York: Human Sciences.

Grieger, R., & Boyd, J. (1980). *Rational-emotive therapy: A skills-based approach*. New York: Van Nostrand Reinhold.

Grieger, R., & Grieger, I (eds.) (1982). *Cognition and emotional disturbance*. New York: Human Sciences Press.

Guidano, K. F. (1988). A systems process-oriented approach to cognitive therapy. In Dobson K. F. (ed.). *Handbook of cognitive-behavioral therapies* (pp. 307–354). New York: Guilford.

Guidano, V. F., & Liotti, G. (1983). *Cognitive processes and emotional disorders*. New York: Guilford.

Haaga, D., & Davison, G. C. (1989). Outcome studies of rational-emotive therapy. In M. E. Bernard & R. A. DiGiuseppe (eds.). *Inside rational-emotive therapy*. San Diego, CA: Acaemic Press.

Haley, Jay. (1976). *Problem solving therapy*. San Francisco: Jossey-Bass.

Harper, R. A. (1960). Marriage counseling as rational process-oriented psychotherapy. *Journal of Individual Psychology, 16*, 197–207.

Harper, R. A. (1981). Limitations of marriage and family therapy. *Rational Living, 16*(2), 3–6.

Hauck, P. A. (1977). *Marriage is a loving business*. Philadelphia: Westminster.

Hauck, P. A. (1980). *Brief counseling with RET*. Philadelphia: Westminster.

Hauck, P. A. (1981). *Overcoming jealousy and possessiveness*. Philadelphia: Westminster.

Hauck, P. A. (1984). *The three faces of love*. Philadelphia: Westminster.

Hayek, F. A. (1978). *New studies in philosophy*. Chicago: University of Chicago Press.

Homans, C. G. (1961). *Social behavior: Its elementary forms*. New York: Harcourt Brace & World.

Huber, C., & Baruth, L. (1989). *Rational-emotive family therapy*. New York: Springer.

Jacobson, N. S., & Margolin, G. (1979). *Marital therapy*. New York: Brunner/Mazel.

Kanfer, F. H., & Schefft, B. K. (1988). *Guiding the process of therapeutic change*. Champaign, IL: Research Press.

Kelly, G. (1955). *The psychology of personal constructs*, 2 vols. New York: Norton.

Kohut, H. (1971). *The analysis of self*, New York: International Universities Press.

Kohut, H. (1977). *The restoration of the self*. New York: International Universities Press.

Korzybski, A. (1933). *Science and sanity*. San Francisco: International Society of General Semantics.

Lange, A., & Jakubowski, P. (1976). *Responsible assertive behavior*. Champaign, IL: Research Press.

Lazarus, A. A. (ed). (1976). *Multimodal behavior therapy*. New York: Springer.

Lazarus, A. A. (1981). *The practice of multimodal therapy*. New York: McGraw-Hill.

Lazarus, A. A. (1985). *Marital myths*. San Luis Obispo, CA: Impact.

Lazarus, R. S. (1982). Thoughts on the relations between emotion and cognition. *American Psychologist, 37*, 1019–1024.

Lazarus, R. S. (1984). On the primacy of cognition. *American Psychologist, 39*, 124–129.

Lederer, W. J., & Jackson, D. D. (1968). *The mirages of marriage*. New York: Norton.

Mahoney, M. J. (1988). *The cognitive sciences and psychotherapy*. In K. S. Dobson (ed.), Handbook of cognitive-behavioral therapies (pp. 357–386). New York: Guilford.

Masters, W., & Johnson, V. A. (1970). *Human sexual inadequacy*. Boston: Little, Brown.

Maultsby, M. C., Jr. (1975). *Help yourself to happiness*. New York: Institute for Rational-Emotive Therapy.

Maultsby, M. C., Jr. (1984). *Rational behavior therapy*. Englewood Cliffs, NJ: Prentice Hall.

Maultsby, M. C., Jr., & Ellis, A. (1974). *Technique for using rational-emotive imagery*. New York: Institute for Rational-Emotive Therapy.

McGovern, T. E., & Silverman, M. S. (1984). A review of outcome studies of rational-emotive therapy from 1977 to 1984. *Journal of Rational-Emotive Therapy*, 2(1), 7–18.

McMullin, R. (1986). *Handbook of cognitive therapy techinques*. New York: Norton.

Meichenbaum, D. (1977). *Cognitive-behavior modification*. New York: Plenum.

Peele, Stanton. (1976). *Love and addiction*. New York: New American Library.

Reda, M. A., & Mahoney, M. J. (Eds.), (1984) *Cognitive psychotherapies*. Cambridge,MA: Ballinger.

Rogers, C. R. (1961). *On becoming a person*. Boston: Houghton-Mifflin.

Rorer, L. T. (in press). Rational-emotive theory: 1. An integrated psychological and philosophical basis. *Cognitive Therapy and Research*.

Russianoff, P. (1982). *Why do I think I am nothing without a man?* New York: Bantam.

Sager, C. J. (1976). *Marriage contracts and marital therapy*. New York: Brunner/Mazel.

Scheflen, A., & Ferber, A. (1972). Critique of a sacred cow. In A. Ferber, M. Mendelsohn, & A. Napier (eds.). *The book of family therapy*. New York: Science House.

Sichel, J., & Ellis, A. (1984). *RET self-help form*. New York: Institute for Rational-Emotive Therapy.

Skinner, B. F. (1953). *Science and human behavior*. New York: Macmillan.

Skinner, B. F. (1971). *Beyond freedom and dignity*. New York: Knopf.

Spivack, G., Platt, J., & Shure, M. (1976). *The problem-solving approach to adjustment*. San Francisco: Jossey-Bass.

Stuart, R. B. (1980). *Helping couples change: A social learning approach to marital therapy*. New York: Guilford.

Tennov, D. (1979). *Love and limerence*. New York: Stein & Day.

Velten, E. (1987). (Speaker). *How to be unhappy at work*, cassette recording. New York: Institute for Rational-Emotive Therapy.

Walen, S. (1985). Rational Sexuality: Some new perspectives. In A. Ellis & M. E. Bernard (eds.), *Clinical aplications of rational-emotive therapy* (pp. 129–152). New York: Plenum.

Walen, S., & Bass, B. (1986). Rational-emotive treatment for the sexual problems of couples. *Journal of Rational-Emotive Therapy*, 4, 82–94.

Walen, S. R., DiGuiseppe, R., & Wessler, R. L. (1980). *A practitioner's guide to rational-emotive therapy*. New York: Oxford.

Wanderer, Z., & Cabot, T. (1978). *Letting go*. New York: Putnam.

Wells, R. A. (1980). Engagement techniques infamily therapy. *International Journal of Family Therapy*, 2(2), 75–94.

Wessler, R. A., & Wessler, R. L. (1980). *The principles and practice of rational-emotive therapy*. San Francisco, CA: Jossey-Bass.

Wolfe, J. L. (Speaker). (1974). *Rational-emotive therapy and women's assertiveness training*, cassette recording. New York: Institute for Rational-Emotive Therapy.

Wolfe, J. L. (Speaker). (1977). *Assertiveness training for women*, cassette recording. New York: BMA Audio Cassettes.

Wolfe, J. L., & Brand, E. (eds.). (1977). *Twenty years of rational therapy*. New York: Institute for Rational-Emotive Therapy.

Wolfe, J. L., & Fodor, I. G. (1975). A cognitive-behavioral approach to modifying assertive behavior in women. *Counseling Psychologist*, 5(4), 45–52.

Young, H. S. (1974). *A rational counseling primer*. New York: Institute for Rational-Emotive Therapy.

Young, H. S. (1984). Special issue: The work of Howard S. Young. *British Journal of Cognitive Psychotherapy, 2*(2), 1–101.

Zajonc, R. B. (1980). Feeling and thinking: Preferences need no inferences. *American Psychologist, 35,* 151–175.

Zajonc, R. B. (1984). On the primacy of affect. *American Psychologist, 39,* 117–123.

Zilbergeld, B. (1978). *Male sexuality.* New York: Bantam.

Author Index

Subject Index

About the Authors

Albert Ellis, Ph.D., is a well-known clinical psychologist, is the founder and president of the Institute for Rational-Emotive Therapy in New York, has practiced marriage and family therapy, sex therapy, and psychotherapy for 46 years, and has published more than 50 books and 600 articles on psychological topics.

Joyce L. Sichel, Ph.D. is a clinical psychologist in practice in Dallas, Texas. She has directed the Rational Living Institute there, and is also on the consulting staff of the public school district and a rehabilitation hospital. She holds degrees from Cornell University, Vassar College, City University of New York, and New York University, and is a Graduate Fellow of the Institute for Rational-Emotive Therapy in New York.

Raymond J. Yeager, Ph.D. is a licensed clinical psychologist in private practice in Huntington and Commack, New York, is Director of Psychological Services at Apple Inc., and is a staff psychologist, supervisor, and member of the training faculty of the Institute for Rational-Emotive Therapy in New York. He has also co-authored *Rational-Emotive Therapy With Alcoholics and Substance Abusers* and *Why Some Therapies Don't Work: The Dangers of Transpersonal Psychology*.

Dominic J. DiMattia, Ed.D. is Hubbell Professor of Counseling, University of Bridgeport and Director of Corporate Services and Staff Therapist at the Institute for Rational-Emotive Therapy in New York. He is a Connecticut Certified Marriage and Family Therapist and author of numerous professional articles.

Raymond DiGiuseppe, Ph.D. is Director of Research and Training at the Institute for Rational-Emotive Therapy in New York and Associate Professor of Psychology at St. Johns University in Jamaica, NY. He is the author of a number of professional articles and co-author of *A Practitioner's Guide to Rational-Emotive Therapy*, *Rational-Emotive Therapy With Alcoholics and Substance Abusers, and Inside Rational-Emotive Therapy*.

Psychology Practitioner Guidebooks

Editors
Arnold P. Goldstein, Syracuse University
Leonard Krasner, Stanford University & SUNY at Stony Brook
Sol L. Garfield, Washington University in St. Louis

William L. Golden, E. Thomas Dowd & Fred Friedberg—
HYPNOTHERAPY: A Modern Approach

Patricia Lacks—BEHAVIORAL TREATMENT FOR PERSISTENT
INSOMNIA

Arnold P. Goldstein & Harold Keller—AGGRESSIVE BEHAVIOR:
Assessment and Intervention

C. Eugene Walker, Barbara L. Bonner & Keith L. Kaufman—
THE PHYSICALLY AND SEXUALLY ABUSED CHILD: Evaluation
and Treatment

Robert E. Becker, Richard G. Heimberg & Alan S. Bellack—SOCIAL
SKILLS TRAINING TREATMENT FOR DEPRESSION

Richard F. Dangel & Richard A. Polster—TEACHING CHILD
MANAGEMENT SKILLS

Albert Ellis, John F. McInerney, Raymond DiGiuseppe & Raymond
Yeager—RATIONAL-EMOTIVE THERAPY WITH ALCOHOLICS
AND SUBSTANCE ABUSERS

Johnny L. Matson & Thomas H. Ollendick—ENHANCING CHILDREN'S
SOCIAL SKILLS: Assessment and Training

Edward B. Blanchard, John E. Martin & Patricia M. Dubbert—NON-DRUG
TREATMENTS FOR ESSENTIAL HYPERTENSION

Samuel M. Turner & Deborah C. Beidel—TREATING OBSESSIVE-
COMPULSIVE DISORDER

Alice W. Pope, Susan M. McHale & W. Edward Craighead—SELF-
ESTEEM ENHANCEMENT WITH CHILDREN AND ADOLESCENTS

Jean E. Rhodes & Leonard A. Jason—PREVENTING SUBSTANCE
ABUSE AMONG CHILDREN AND ADOLESCENTS

Gerald D. Oster, Janice E. Caro, Daniel R. Eagen & Margaret A. Lillo—
ASSESSING ADOLESCENTS

Robin C. Winkler, Dirck W. Brown, Margaret van Keppel & Amy
Blanchard—CLINICAL PRACTICE IN ADOPTION

Roger Poppen—BEHAVIORAL RELAXATION TRAINING AND
ASSESSMENT

Michael D. LeBow—ADULT OBESITY THERAPY

Robert Paul Liberman, William J. DeRisi & Kim T. Mueser—SOCIAL
SKILLS TRAINING FOR PSYCHIATRIC PATIENTS

Johnny L. Matson—TREATING DEPRESSION IN CHILDREN AND
ADOLESCENTS

Sol L. Garfield—THE PRACTICE OF BRIEF PSYCHOTHERAPY

Arnold P. Goldstein, Barry Glick, Mary Jane Irwin,
Claudia Pask-McCartney & Ibrahim Rubama—REDUCING
DELINQUENCY: Intervention in the Community

Albert Ellis, Joyce L. Sichel, Raymond J. Yeager, Dominic J. DiMattia,
Raymond DiGiuseppe—RATIONAL-EMOTIVE COUPLES THERAPY